WOMEN'S HEALTH IN THE COMMUNITY

SERIES EDITOR
June Clark PhD BA MPhil SRN HVCert

In the Same Series

Professional Responsibility
Health Education — Practical Teaching Techniques
Counselling and the Nurse — An Introduction
Hard-to-Help Families
Infant Feeding and Family Nutrition
The Nurse and the Welfare State
Multiple Births
Dying at Home
British Asians — Health Care in the Community

TOPICS IN COMMUNITY HEALTH Series

WOMEN'S HEALTH IN THE COMMUNITY

Edited by

JEAN ORR MSc BA SRN HVT CertEd
Lecturer, Department of Nursing
Victoria University of Manchester

With 12 Contributors

An H M + M Nursing Publication

JOHN WILEY & SONS
Chichester · New York · Brisbane · Toronto · Singapore

Copyright © 1987 by John Wiley & Sons Ltd

All rights reserved

No part of this book may be reproduced by any
means, or transmitted, or translated into
a machine language without the written
permission of the publisher.

H M + M is an imprint of John Wiley & Sons Ltd,
Baffins Lane, Chichester, Sussex, England

British Library Cataloguing in Publication Data:

Women's health in the community — (Topics
 in community health) — (An HM+M nursing
 publication)
 1. Women's health services — Great Britain
 I. Orr, Jean II. Series
 362.1'98'0941   RA564.85

ISBN 0 471 91105 4

Library of Congress Cataloging-in-Publication Data:

Women's health in the community.

 (Topics in community health) (An HM+M nursing
publication)
  Includes index.
  1. Women's health services — Great Britain.
2. Community health services — Great Britain. I. Orr,
Jean. II. Series. III. Series: An HM+M nursing
publication. [DNLM: 1. Community Health Services —
Great Britain. WA 546 FA1 W8]
RA564.85.W68 1987   362.1'98'0941   86-32485
ISBN 0 471 91105 4

Printed and bound in Great Britain

DEDICATION

We dedicate this book to the memory of Judith Gray. We were privileged to know her as a woman, a friend, a feminist, a doctor, and as a campaigner for peace and the women's health movement.

CONTENTS

	Introduction – *Jean Orr*	1
1	Health/Illness in Healing/Caring – A Feminist Perspective – *Margaret Ann O'Connor*	5
2	Making Sense of Feminist Contributions to Women's Health – *Anne Williams*	23
3	Defining Women and their Health: The Case of Hysterectomy – *Christine Webb*	39
4	Some of the Issues of Childbirth – *Ann M Thomson*	57
5	Women and Mental Health – *Lorraine Smith*	76
6	The Development of Well Woman Clinics – *Pat Thornley*	97
7	The Manchester Experience I: Wythenshawe Well Woman Clinic – *Rebekah Williams*	107
8	The Manchester Experience II: Withington Well Woman Clinic – *Joan Armstrong*	129
9	The Manchester Experience III: Rusholme Well Women Clinic – *Claire Ronalds*	138
10	The Liverpool Experience: The Croxteth Women's Health Group: Self-help on a Deprived Community of Liverpool – *Effie Sherlock*	153
11	Economic Aspects of Women's Health – *Wendy Hull*	167
	In Conclusion – *Jean Orr*	181

| Appendix: Well Woman Clinic Questionnaire | 187 |
| Index | 199 |

PREFACE

The rise of the women's health movement over the past four or five years has been a major innovatory feature of community health care in the United Kingdom, and it is appropriate that an analysis and description of this movement should be made available to a wide range of health workers, including health visitors, district nurses, community health workers, health education officers and workers from many voluntary organisations. Thus this book is intended to furnish a critique of the well woman movement and the implications for women as providers as well as receivers of health care.

In this volume the historical, political and economic aspects of women's health are described and discussed from a feminist perspective, and issues such as the control of women by nurses and alternative health care for women, which up to now have been largely ignored, are also addressed. Its features include a considerable range of case study material on the implementation and organisation of well woman clinics and the implications such clinics have for existing health care services. This book will be of interest to students of social policy and students on the many courses which have a focus on women's issues.

JEAN ORR
Manchester 1987

CONTRIBUTORS

JOAN ARMSTRONG   Nursing Officer, South Manchester District

MERRYN COOKE   Counsellor, Rusholme Health Centre, Manchester

WENDY HULL   Formerly Deputy Treasurer, Harrow Health District; Lecturer for Accounting, Centre for Health Planning and Management, Keele University

MARGARET O'CONNOR   Lecturer in Health Visiting, Mid-Kent College of Higher and Further Education

JEAN ORR   Lecturer in Nursing, University of Manchester

CLARE RONALDS   General Practitioner, Rusholme Health Centre, Manchester

EFFIE SHERLOCK   Health Education Worker, Manchester

LORRAINE SMITH   Lecturer in Nursing, University of Manchester

ANN M THOMSON   Clinical Lecturer, University of Manchester

PAT THORNLEY   Lay Health Worker, Liverpool

CHRISTINE WEBB   Principal Lecturer, Department of Nursing, Health and Applied Social Studies, Bristol Polytechnic

ANNE WILLIAMS   Part-time Lecturer, Department of Social Administration, University of Lancaster

REBEKAH WILLIAMS   Research Psychologist, Manchester Royal Infirmary

INTRODUCTION

Jean Orr

This book is a result of women coming together to record their perceptions, experiences and commitment to the women's health movement. We come from different backgrounds of nursing, health visiting, midwifery, medicine, economics and social sciences. Some of us are teachers, other are practitioners and researchers. Although all of us may not call ourselves feminists we are united in our concern for women and in the provision of services which best meet their needs. Many of the contributors were involved in the early days of this movement in the North-West of England and helped to translate grass-roots demand for change into action. Those of us involved found it exciting and challenging to see women breaking the stereotypes of class and sex. For too long it was said that women, particularly working-class women, would not or could not organise and articulate their demands. We saw that women could come together and express their dissatisfaction with existing services and exert pressure to influence health care policy.

Women started campaigns for well woman clinics and health courses, often independent of the professionals. They demanded services which best met their needs and which by definition were critical of existing services. There is an inherent difficulty for professionals in this type of criticism no matter how much they sympathise with the aim of their critics. It takes a shift in professional/client perspectives and in the professional/lay worker relationship. Like all change it is not easy. The women's health movement is linked to the re-emergence of feminism in 1960/1970. The growing body of feminist literature identifies women's issues in relation to health care and provides insights about women's role which are crucial to those providing health care. One does not need to be a feminist in order to recognise that women's experiences have been devalued and denied. There is very little emphasis given to any critical examination of women's health in professional education. This is true even in the preparation of workers who work primarily with women, e.g. health visitors and midwives.

Nurses are one group of workers who should be most concerned about women's health issues, both as providers and recipients of the service. Women take most responsibility for the maintenance of family health in terms of nutrition, safety and nursing of family members. On the one hand mothers/ women are seen to be the lynch pin of family life but on the other there is little emphasis on their health outside their reproductive role, and this is often as a means of control.

This book has three main themes, moving from general issues to the particular examples of well women clinics. We start by looking at the relationship between feminism and health care, move on to discuss three issues of particular, relevance to women's health, before examining the setting up and running of well woman clinics. The earlier chapters inform and set in context the processes which led to the establishment of the clinics.

Margaret O'Connor explores women's health from a feminist perspective, drawing on historical and philosophical evidence to illustrate and explain present day services. Much of the feminist writing helps us to see that the personal concerns of women can become political, and Anne Williams explores how her understanding of feminism has developed through her reading of feminist literature in the health field.

In the second theme we move to examine three health issues which are of particular relevance to women. Christine Webb shows how psychological theories have been used to define women when they are healthy and when they are sick and uses the example of hysterectomy to illustrate the process of categorising women as being ruled by their psychology and emotions. Ann Thomson, in her writing on some of the issues in childbirth, raises questions on how social and economic factors effect the outcome of pregnancy. Lorraine Smith examines the area of mental health, looking at role-conflict for women and its accompanying experience of stress. She discusses the theme of loss in women's life and suggests various coping mechanisms to help women change and gain control of their lives.

The third theme in the book concentrates on well woman clinics. Pat Thornley traces the development of how different models of well woman clinics have formed and explores the reasons underpinning their rationale. Rebekah Williams discusses the South Manchester Clinics by documenting the series of events and basic philosophy surrounding the setting up of a clinic and the benefits gained by lay and professional people working together: it is a case study of effecting change. Joan Armstrong writes about the Withington Clinic and Clare Ronalds and Merryn Cooke describe a clinic in Rusholme Health Centre. Effie Sherlock describes her involvement with a self-help women's group in Liverpool.

These contributors show that there is no one model of a well woman clinic and that each group of workers create services which meet local demand and circumstances. To make the case for policy changes is never easy and Wendy Hull looks at some of the economic issues surrounding allocation of resources and suggests ways to make a case to policy makers.

The main reason why we are interested in promoting women's health is because women have a right to achieve their optimum level of wellness. While recognising the social and economic influences on health we can encourage them to be responsible for their own well being by helping them to increase their self esteem. Traditionally, concern about women's health has been justified in terms of their role within the family as the main care giver and the 'producer' of future generations. This has been the impetus for much of health care policy and as such it has been limited and controlling. The women's health movement while recognising the reality of women's reproductive and nurturing functions takes a much broader view of women's lives and makes legitimate demands for services which meet the needs of the 'whole woman' irrespective of age or social status.

Chapter 1

HEALTH/ILLNESS IN HEALING/CARING – A FEMINIST PERSPECTIVE

Margaret Ann O'Connor

'The dominant sex is embedded in the dominant institutional position with respect to health care.' (Navarro 1979)

The notion that health is closely linked to the theory and practice of medicine has implications for women in terms of their health care and roles as health carers. Feminists regard medical knowledge as part of the means by which gender divisions in society are maintained. Medicine does not merely reflect the discriminatory views of women held by society, but serves to reproduce these views by actively creating stereotypes and controlling women who deviate from them (Doyal 1983). This genderised concept of medicine/health needs, needs to be examined in terms of ideologies that are inculcated into the medical paradigm and the effect on women clients/patients and female professionals. In this chapter the historical and philosophical antecedents and their impact on health care today will be examined from a feminist perspective.

History

Before the Industrial Revolution women undertook a wide variety of productive activity. The home was the centre of production and consumption, there was no sharp division between the private close relationship notion of the home which is geared to reproduction and consumption, and the public arena, in which individuals act out productive work roles. In the old order, men and women had clearly defined but complementary roles (Doyal 1983). Whilst the menfolk were outside the home hunting for food, it was the women elders who cared for the sick and used herbal remedies. It was the women who bore children themselves who became the midwives (Ehrenreich & English 1979). Essentially, with the exception of obstetrics and gynaecology, women were viewed as having the same health needs as men. Soranus (28–138 AD) summarises the views of these early writers on health and illness.

'Female has her illness in common with the male, she suffers from constriction or from flux either acutely or chronically, and she is subject to the same seasonal differences, to graduations of disease, to lack of strength, and to the different foreign bodies, sores and injuries. Only as far as particulars and specific variations are concerned does the female show conditions peculiarly her own, ie. a different character of symptoms. Therefore, she is subject to treatment generically the same.' (Quoted by Marieskind 1980, p 2).

Up to the 12th century, women healers were found in all levels of society. The early priestess-physicians carried out midwifery, public health work, hospital administration, herbal cures, some dentistry and surgery as well as medical education. (Marieskind 1980). The establishment of the universities in the 13th century prevented the admission of women to higher education and, subsequently, medicine. The Church, State and social convention collectively were used by physicians to exclude women from their ranks. The Law was used to prevent the literate woman healers from practising. In 1421 petitions were sent to Henry V bewailing 'the presumptions of women who undermine the profession' and asked that 'no woman use the practice of fisyk under payne of long imprisonment' (Jones I B, quoted by Marieskind, p 118). Thus, whilst the female lay healer 'operated a network of information sharing and mutual support, the male professional horded up his knowledge as a kind of property'. (Ehrenreich & English 1979, p 66). The female lay healer was in fact antithetical to the male medical professional.

The alliance between Church, State and the universities led to the rise of the medical profession, to an elitist system which not only isolated women but led to practices which established the security of their position. The campaign of the physician against the great mass of women healers was conducted by the

Church. It was the Church that denounced non-professional healing as heresy, 'If a woman dare to cure without having studied she is a witch and must die' (Ehrenreich & English 1979, p 35). Thus, the male physician was placed on a higher moral and intellectual plain whilst the woman healer, the witch, was placed on the side of darkness evil and magic (Ibid).

Women healers who used charms as well as herbs were seen as carrying out evil practices; whilst the activities of the physician (who was educated in theology, not medicine), such as bleeding, cupping and administering potions made from black snake skins, etc., were seen as bone fide.

By the 15th and 16th centuries, witchhunts and executions were endemic in Europe. The midwives suffered greatly at the hands of their inquisitors. 'The greatest injuries to the Faith as regards the heresy of witches are done by midwives, and this is made clearer than daylight itself by the confessions of some who were afterwards burned' (Kramer & Sprenger 1968). Nevertheless, midwifery survived.

Some outstanding midwives were to be found among those practising in the 17th and 18th centuries. Jane Sharpe wrote *The Compleate Midwive's Companion* in (1671) in which she strongly advised midwives to study anatomy. She defended midwives against male domination, stating that 'the art of midwifery chiefly concerns us (women) which even the best learned men will grant . . They are forced to borrow from us the very name they practice by . . . man midwives' (Jex-Blake 1886, p 17–19). Many other midwives, ie. Mrs Cellier (1687) and Mrs Elizabeth Nihell (1723), continued to attack the practice of the rising number of man midwives. These women used mortality and morbidity statistics to emphasise the need for proper care and facilities for mothers and babies. They vehemently attacked the male obstetric practices of the day. Elizabeth Nihell called William Smellie (1697–1763) a 'great horse godmother of a he midwife'. She abhorred his practice of allowing his novice male obstetricians to treat charity patients. She described it as 'the work of two or three maggots (who) have produced thousands of . . . novices who watch the distress of poor pregnant women, . . . they make these poor wretches, hired for their purpose, undergo the most inhuman vexation' (Findley 1939). Men midwives were also strong advocates of lying-in hospitals which served to increase puerperal sepsis and the infant and maternal mortality rates. 'Virtually until this century, women in labour could only hope that harm would not be done to them, and midwives in general were probably less harmful than men' (Leeson & Gray 1978, p 54).

Philosophy

Philosophical ideas of the 17th and 18th centuries were used to define the position of women. The Enlightenment was a period during which the opposition between the nature and the state of society or of education was explored. Rousseau, working on traditions established long before his time, saw the concept of nature as being crucial to his radical advocacy of sovereignty of people and the legitimacy of democracy (MacCormack 1980). However, these 18th-century ideas did not extend to women. These philosophies accepted the traditional view that woman was closer to nature than man because of her physiological role in sex and motherhood. Nature was associated with romantic notions of women's emotions and domesticity. Women were seen as the repositories of natural law – the founder of human society was the mother of the family. Nature could therefore be revealed and understood through the scientific unveiling of women (Jordanova 1980). At the same time, women were also the repositories of passions which needed to be contained and controlled. By the mid-18th century the well-established biomedical tradition observed and defined humans in terms of conceptual divisions between unique female and unique male attributes. 'A biological determinism explained women, but men were defined by their social acts' (MacCormack 1980, p 21).

This assumption that women were closer to nature took many forms. The German philosopher Stahl held that the soul's purpose was to preserve the body in order to achieve its own goal of mental activity. In women however, this purpose of the soul was subordinate to motherhood. It was through the continuation of the species that women's goal of mental activity would be achieved. For Stahl, woman was more stable than man. She was governed by three fundamental affections:

'(i) Pleasure which corresponds to her need to be impregnated.
(ii) Fear which ensures care of the embryo.
(iii) Inconstancy because she must be able to dispense affection to all the children she conceives. She unconsciously and spon-

taneously chooses a quiet protected life which is suited to her ultimate purpose of procreation' (Bloch & Bloch 1980, p 33).

The dichotomy between women as nature and men as culture, reinforced the division between the public (work) and the private (home). These ideas enabled such writers as Michelet to cite marriage as an ideal moral state in which each partner was the moral guardian of the other. Women who worked outside the home, and men who refused to marry were seen as impediments to this ideal. On the one hand, romanticism saw women as home makers, the providers of an idyllic refuge from the unpleasant world of men; (Ehrenreich & English 1979); on the other hand, private workers were seen as conservative against political change and having a vested interest in maintaining traditional views, ie. of the Church, etc. (Jordanova 1980).

This association of women with the romantic tradition of nature and men with culture and rational thought, ensured that women were deemed to be incapable of analytical thought. Hence, the ideology of progress entrenched in enlightenment thought such as the growth of a humane rational and civilised society, established the domination of male value systems on the female.

These ideas were taught and developed by Dr Roussel in France who argued that it would be wrong for women to engage in intellectual activity. 'Let women leave to men the doubtful benefit that they seek in this dangerous enterprise (intellectual work): nature has done enough for them already and it would be an offence against her if through such activity women were to lose the centre of precious gifts which she has bestowed'. (Block & Block 1980, p 33). The early specialists in psychology ensured that womans intellectual capabilities were linked to her reproductive capacities. Dr Hall denied educational opportunities to many girls on the grounds that it would weaken her productive organs. Female functions such as menstruation were used to validate severe limitations to intellectual opportunity; girls, therefore, received education in domestic crafts, the arts and needlework (Doyal 1981, p 100).

Medical hegemony in the 19th century

By the 19th century women were expected to conform to the sexual romanticist ideal of femininity. Marriage was a sexual economic relationship in which women performed sexual and reproductive duties for financial support. 'A successful man could have no better social ornament than an idle wife. Her delicacy, her culture, her child-like ignorance of the male could give a man class which money could not buy' (Ehrenreich & English 1979, p 95). This position subjected women to lives of boring idleness which was often associated with sickness. This sickness in turn legitimised a life of idleness. Hence, upper class women became the legitimate subjects of the rising male physician. This myth of female frailty and hypochondria served to disqualify women as healers and made women highly qualified as patients. Also the association of women with idleness/sickness ensured the sexual division of labour within the middle classes. It arose at the same time that health/medical care was being recast as a commodity within the framework of a capitalist economy. The medical profession therefore, had most contact with rich bourgeois women, bourgeois woman thereby became ideal woman. Working class women were seen as being of different stock and therefore able to work without risking their health.

Despite opposition from the Popular Health Movement, working-class and women's movements of the early 19th Century (McLauren 1977; Woodward & Richards 1977), biological determinism and philosophical notions of natural roles served to give ideological justification in terms of health and illness, diagnosis and treatment, to the medical profession. Further, evolutionary and psychological theories reflected the capitalist economy whereby men became the producers and specialists, whilst women were differentiated according to their reproductive capacities as wives and mothers. Medical focus on female disease served to emphasise sexual difference. Within the medical model, the uterus was seen as the controlling organ with woman built around it. (Ehrenreich & English, 1979, p 108) Physicians and specialists served to widen the distinction between sexuality and reproduction. Whilst the reproductive functions of women were emphasised, female sexuality was seen as abnormally detrimental. The uterus and ovaries were blamed for disorders, the most common intervention being ovariectomy. The historian Barker-Benfield documented the reasons for such drastic surgical intervention: 'Among the indications were troublesomeness, eating like a ploughman masturbation, attempted suicide, erotic tendencies, persecution mania, simple "cussedness", and dysmenorrhoea. Most apparent, in the enormous variety of symptoms doctors took to indicate castration was a strong current of sexual appetitiveness on the part of women.' (Quoted by Ehrenreich & English 1979, p 111).

Medical discoveries of micro-organisms linked to the need for domestic cleanliness were encompassed within notions of domestic science. The discovery of the child and the 'science' of child psychology led to further entrenchment of women as domestic workers and mothers. This scientific approach towards domestic health and child care was welcomed by many early feminists who felt that science would elevate the status of women's work within the home (Ehrenreich & English 1979). However, such theories were used to expand the domestic duties and ties of women within the private arena, thus widening the gulf between the private and public spheres. When women expressed dissatisfaction with their lot, malfunctioning reproductive organs were blamed and were often treated as gynaecological or psychosomatic problems of female sexuality.

Women as Patients/Clients

Freud's theories of female sexuality and the discovery of hormones served to scientficially validate the link between brain and uterus. Also the notion that femininity was pathological laid the way open to medical intervention in that it complied with the tacit belief that men are 'normal' and women are 'abnormal'. Further, this covert belief ensured that, when measured against men, women are essentially defective. The consequences of such ideologies is that women use the health service more than men, ie. women aged between 15–44 years and 65–75 years make far greater use of local medical services. (Hart 1982). Also, women's illnesses are not taken seriously and are not likely to be seen as having a biological cause (Scully 1980).

The higher incidence of women patients suffering from mental illness is due to the acceptance that it is still socially desirable for women to acknowledge symptoms of weakness or stress. Men act out stress through drinking alcohol, smoking, and so on. In women, stress, which is often the outcome of a situation, tends to be labelled mental illness which then requires psychiatric assistance. Mental illness is, therefore, not a distinct disease but the result of a series of events which ends in definitions by social control agencies (Smith 1975). It is a process whereby male psychiatrists control the behaviour of different sexes on different criteria (Clarke 1983). Further, the use of psychotrophic drugs by doctors helps them to see women's problems as 'unreal'. This notion is illustrated by Barbara's (a member of a well women's group) description of womens experiences. 'When they (women) went to their doctor for menopausal problems they got handed tranquillisers, no attempt was made to advise on the menopause. There seemed to be a tendency for a lot of doctors to deal with specific female complaints with handouts in the form of tranquillisers, when women wanted more advice, more authoritative and practical help '(O'Connor 1984, p 59). Tranquillisers also have a social meaning in that they show how women use mood altering drugs to help them cope with unsatisfactory lives and relationships, roles and relationships which are structurally determined (Cooperstock & Leonard 1979). This medical perception of the unreality of women's conditions extends to other conditions such as dysmenorrhea, pain of labour, nausea of pregnancy and behaviour disturbances which are considered to be caused or aggravated by psychogenic facts. Although scientific evidence indicates that they may be organic causes, 'acceptance of a psychogenic origin has led to irrational and ineffective approach to their management' (Leanne & Leanne 1973).

Surgical intervention in women's conditions is also significant. In the USA in the years 1975 and 1976, women experienced 63% of all surgical operations. In the 15–44 age group, women had 2½ times more operations than men in the same age group. Much of this was sex specific, eg. D & Cs, hysterectomies (Scully 1980). In Britain, the rate of surgical intervention in the genital organs is 3½ times more numerous in women than men. This may be partly due to the fact that there is no male medical speciality that is equivalent to gynaecology.

Further, medical effort is not just concerned with disease: 'As guardians of the process of human reproduction, doctors are responsible for regulating the supply of female contraception and for supervising childbirth' (Hart 1982).

Graham & Oakley (1981) have traced the medicalisation of

normal reproduction and the conflict that this engenders between women and the medical profession in obstetric care. They describe the obstetrician's frame of reference which attaches a particular and limited significance to pregnancy and birth as medical events. 'The doctor views the individuals career as a pregnant and parturant woman as an isolated patient episode'. The mother however, sees reproduction not as an isolated episode of medical treatment but as an event which is integrated with other aspects of her life. 'Having a baby affects not only her medical status, it has implications for most of her social roles . . . her pregnancy affects her occupational standing, her financial position, her housing situation, her marital status and her personal relationships'. By using medical technology, professionals and institutions in the reproductive services have relocated pregnancy within the bounds of the medical paradigm and thus redefined normal confinement as an illness. This unequal relationship between the mother and doctor results in isolation of pregnant women, and the maintenance of ignorance of the mother. Hence, the pregnant woman is unable to take full part in her own pregnancy and birth.

Control of the reproductive capacities of women by women is regarded as the main means whereby women's health can be improved and women liberated. Since it is men who control the Church, State, medical profession and drug companies, it is men who define and control the moral/legal sanctions and the production and distribution of forms of birth control. For women, the most effective forms of birth control can only be obtained through the medical profession. Research into birth control is made to fit into male defined categories. It is women, not men, who are exposed to the side effects of the systemic contraceptive pill, interuterine device, and so on (Roberts 1981).

Women as Health Workers

The ideology of the reproductive nature of femininity has also been at work in the job market. The notion of 'women's work is in the home' which arose during the Industrial Revolution widened the division between the private (domestic) and public (workplace). This biological determinant/domestic service image of women's work, and the patriachal tradition in the division of labour, placed limitations on the jobs that were available to women. In 1898

19% women were in domestic service.

26% were garment makers

14% were textile workers

these jobs were classified as low-status and were low-paid (Doyal 1981, p 151).

At the turn of the century women in the 20 – 35 year group outnumbered men and therefore had fewer chances of marriage. For these 'surplus women' it was economically imperative that they should find work. Such jobs as teaching and nursing, were seen as distinctly women's work (Magg 1984, p 32).

Biological and moral ideologies were used to define nursing as essentially women's work. The ability to care for the helpless was seen as women's 'distinctive nature'. 'Nursing is mothering grown up folks when sick, all are babies' (Muff 1982, p 104). Indeed, visits by health visitors in the 19th Century served to locate middle class individualistic notions of motherhood onto working class women (Davin 1978). Nursing was also seen as being eminently suitable in terms of womens socialisation roles as wives since it ensured obedience to the physician's orders. Florence Nightingale complied with this; 'Never assert your opinions and wishes but defer to his you will find that in the end, you generally have your own way. This is a truly feminine piece of counsel and I beg you to lay it on your heart' (*The Hospital*, 8 January 1898, p 127). This paternalistic stereotype of the nurse served to reinforce the idea that nurses lack intelligence, autonomy and tended to ensure female nurses' passive behaviour.

The structure of the NHS reflects the class structure of the capitalist society in that its labour force is specialist, stratified, each level having differing pay, status and power over work. It is also divided in terms of gender and race. Most doctors are from middle class backgrounds and are male. Approximately 75% of the workforce in the NHS are women and most of them carry out domestic caring tasks, and are not represented at higher levels. Most women at the lowest levels are black (Doyal 1981).

Even when women are admitted to medicine they are outnumbered by men (27% of doctors are women), and they are subject to a patriarchal ideology that permeates all medical institutions. Linda Grant's (1983) research into sexism in medical education highlights the importance of the peer group as unconscious 'social mirrors' of this ideology. She endeavoured to test the hypothesis that women experience conflict about female identity when they compete with men in an area defined as masculine, and that this conflict is expressed in a lowering and devaluation of aspirations/competences as well as a motivation to avoid success. Her analysis of male and female medical students, peer group and self assessments showed that men were highly rated by themselves and their peers, as instructors, researchers in medical science and in knowledge of medical science. Women rated themselves higher in sensitivity to patients and valued happiness at work. A preponderance of male and some female peers overrated women students in the sensitivity dimension. Other researchers endorse this notion of sexism in medical education. Savage & Tate (1983) found that male medical students do not regard women as equals: about one third of their sample from the London Hospital felt that women were more suited to nursing than medicine; one half felt that there should be a restriction on the proportion of women entering medicine.

This ideology is expressed in postgraduate education and is reflected in job opportunities. In general practice many male principals are unwilling to appoint a female partner who may become pregnant (Reynolds 1982). Not only is the woman doctor denied a job because of the stereotype but at the same time, 'the partners may not want to deal with women's clinical problems, so they try to get a woman trainee' (p 69), hence the postgraduate woman trainee is exploited. This form of exploitation also extends to women in general in that a male partner is more likely to be taken on 'especially if he has a wife or girlfriend who lives with him to answer the telephone'. Female doctors are not represented in the prestige specialities of medicine, surgery and obstetrics/gynaecology. They tend to occupy positions in community health, school medicine, family planning, laboratory based specialities, psychiatry, part-time sub consultants posts and part-time general practice assistanceships. The Medical Practitioners Union (1982) cite this distribution of female doctors in the medical services as 'prima facie evidence of discrimination'.

At a time when it is evident that women would prefer women to care for them (Womens National Commission Report 1985; Preston-Whyte *et al.* 1983), nursing is still firmly under the domination of the male medical profession. While on the one hand nursing is being pulled under the hospital medical umbrella away from care towards high technology intervention, on the other hand the previously autonomous role of the community nurse and health visitor is being more and more defined and controlled by the general practitioner. The result of this process of domination is deskilling. Indeed, the recent domination of midwifery is an example. Despite lengthened training, the midwife's role has been reduced to that of a subserviant, fragmented, hospital-based obstetric nurse. Hence, 'The roles that different members of the (health) team play are primarily due to their class background and sex role, and only secondary, very secondary indeed to their technological knowledge' (Navarro 1975, 1 p 361).

Structural attempts to improve the status of nurses within the NHS have not taken into account the needs of a profession in which there is a predominance of women. The imposition of a hierarchical bureaucratic management structure (Salmon) onto the nursing profession has thereby ensured that many nurses remain in low-status, low-paid jobs, whilst the few, who are often men, manage to obtain top management positions.

The need to raise the consciousness of women workers in the NHS is, therefore, of paramount importance to nurses. This can only be done not only through education but through practical facilities ie. crêches and management strategies that take into account the domestic ties of women which militate against their ability to seek promotion. However, the challenge to male domination of the NHS is coming not from within the service but outside it, in the community from the feminist movement.

Community care

In Britain, between 75% and 85% of illness is managed without a doctor's consultation (Levin 1981, p 185). Most of this care is provided by women in the community (WHO 1983); women are therefore not just consumers, but major producers of health. They have always been responsible for the care of people who the NHS will not look after. This domestic work is increasing with demographic changes. During the last 20 years the number of people aged 65 years has increased by one third. There are 3 million people aged over 75 years, most of whom are women (Doyal 1983). This invisibility of the enormous amount of care done by women in the private arena (as well as in the public arena) confirms the asymmetry in the cultural value of male and female, 'male as opposed to female activity is recognised as predominantly important, and cultural systems give authority and value to the roles and activities of men' (Rosaldo 1974, p 19).

Caring is described by psychologists as the means by which women achieve femininity – it is synonymous with notions of self-fulfillment within the roles of wife, mother, daughter (Graham 1983, p 15). Whilst the woman remains economically dependent on her competitive male partner, her role is dependent on her ability to be depended upon as a carer. Therefore, the caring role of the woman is more than universal feelings that women have for family members, it also describes a specific kind of *labour*: 'It is something women do for others to keep them alive. Life is something bartered between carer and cared for' (Graham 1983, p 25).

Caring is seen as having two elements, namely (i) caring *about* (ii) caring *for* (Parker 1980). These two concepts do not have the same emotional basis ie. a person can be cared for without being cared about and vise versa. The *labour* of caring 'describes the direct work which is performed in looking after those who temporarily cannot do for themselves. It comprises such things as feeding, washing, lifting, protecting, representing, comforting' (Ungerson 1983, p 63). These tasks of caring are seen as having much in common with notions of mothering. Ungerson's examination of the appropriateness of the mothering model of care raises questions as to its effectiveness in meeting the needs of the cared for. For her, the mother/child model is inappropriate when extended to the care of the mentally handicapped and elderly since it places them in infantile roles. Whilst some elderly patients/clients in institutions may use this child like status of dependency to manipulate staff, those patients/clients who do not want to shed their independence suffer and are disliked by nursing staff. Within the domestic sphere, the emotional problems that are raised through the reversal of mother/daughter roles can put intolerable pressures on the 'carer' and 'cared for'. 'It is not uncommon in a strict parent-child hierarchy for the parent quite bluntly to refuse to do what the daughter suggests because she maintains, she will not be guided by her child.'

The question that Ungerson raises should perhaps, not concern itself so much with whether the model of mother is appropriate, but *why* the mother/infant relationship is extended to the elderly, the mentally handicapped, and so on. Surely the mothering model also encompasses the facilitation of the growth and development of the child into an independent adult? This aspect of mothering is often mirrored in the nursing care of curable, high-status sick adults. Such patients are the recipients of intensive rehabilatative nursing care. The question it raises is whether forms of mothering, as expressed by nurse/carers, reflects and confirms society's values in that it not only confirms, but controls patient's status. The handicapped/elderly have no economically productive status in society to be rehabilitated into. If the elderly person refuses to give up maternal power to the nurse or daughter, she is labelled disruptive in the institution; in the domestic sphere, the daughter is advised to 'bring the general practitioner, health visitor or social worker into the scene, they will probably tell your mother a few home truths' (McKenzie 1980, p 53).

It appears that forms of mothering are used to control certain patients/clients; at the same time, they are the means whereby female carers are oppressed. On the one hand, the woman's status within the family is dependent upon the dependence of the 'cared for', on the other hand, this role condemns the 'carer' to many years of lonely, isolated, unpaid labour.

Feminist epidemiology

Recent developments in feminist epidemiological studies are beginning to make visible the causes of ill health in women. The predominance of men, ie. male occupations, in official statistics and the lack of documentation of female occupations, has resulted in a failure to recognise and direct preventive strategy to the occupational health needs of women. This skewing of statistics in favour of men, serves to reinforce the stereotype of women as housewives at a time when in fact, 50% of women with dependent children, are working outside the home (Women's National Commission Report 1984). Such problems as dysmenorrhoea due to occupation, infections, sexual harrassment and chemical/radiation hazards, are now being documented or placed on the agenda. Also, health profiles of women in the private arena are being highlighted, ie. the preponderance of violence and accidents suffered by women in the home (Doyal 1983). Feminist health researchers are also compiling a critique of the NHS and other related agencies, ie, they explain that the difficulties of obtaining data on rape, violence, and so on, is due, in part, to the reluctance of women victims to utilise the service of agencies and staff whose behaviour reflect patriachal social mores.

The predominance of male medical/specialist quantitative analysis of health/illness is challenged by feminist epidemiology. Although men's health is deemed to be poorer than women's, since men figure predominantly in mortality statistics, feminist qualitative analysis raises questions as to the meaning of health and illness: whilst the feminist perspective acknowledges that men's lives are short and brutal, it also reveals that women's lives are long and miserable (Hart 1982). Thus, the feminist perspective embraces a broader notion of health/illness and it consciously recognises that the Health Service reflects political, ideological and economic factors in society. The feminist epidemiological approach could be said to represent, not only a paradigm shift from specialist to holistic health care, but also a political basis for an economic and ideological transition from a health care system based on male-dominated market forces, to a more egalitarian community-focused approach to health care.

Conclusion

Patriachal hegemony over the concept of health/illness – healing/caring serves to oppress women both as patients/clients and as health workers/carers. Feminist studies of caring in the public and private spheres, not only highlight the extensive contribution made by women to health care, but also, the interactive processes that serve to remake and confirm sex roles. These studies also focus on the intervention of the State into the public sphere (Finch & Groves 1983; Roberts 1983). The State bridges the dichotomy between the public and the private and, through its policies and laws, confirms sex stereotypes. At the same time, the State (and its institutions) is an arena in which, and through which, sexism can be challenged. Lastly, feminists analysis of caring raises fundamental questions about the ideological basis of nursing care. For some feminists, a more equal division of labour between men and women as carers would benefit both the carers and the cared for. Sensitive research into the deep-seated taboos that place limitations on the caring tasks that men, as opposed to women, do in the home, may elucidate the problem. The feminist perspective demonstrates the needs for nurses to form stronger links with women as providers, and women as users of health care. It is only through such liaison that the extent of women's contribution to health care will be recognised. This would lead to a critical re-evaluation of the beliefs and practices of western scientific medicine, particularly in terms of the low status of caring vis à vis medical intervention, and its relationship with the status of patients/clients.

At a time when the NHS is subject to financial restrictions, and official rhetoric is centred on community care, the implications of such policies for women must be represented and made visible, not only by womens groups in the community, but by female nurses in the National Health Service.

References

Bloch M & Bloch J H (1980) Women and the dialects of Nature in eighteenth century French thought. In MacCormack C & Strathen M (eds) *Nature Culture and Gender*. Cambridge University Press.

Clarke J M (1983) Sexism, feminism and medicalism: a decade review of literature on gender and illness. *Sociology of Health and Illness*, **5** (1), 62–82

Cooperstock R & Lennard H L (1979) Some social meanings of tranquilliser use. *Sociology of Health and Illness*, 3(2), 36–39

Davin A (1978) Imperialism and motherhood. *History Journal Workshop*, **5**, 9–65

Doyal L (1983) Women, health and the sexual division of labour: a case study of the women's health movement in Britain. *International Journal of Health Services*, **13** (3), 373–387

Doyal L & Pennell I (1981) *The Political Economy of Health*. London: Pluto Press

Ehrenreich B & English D (1979) *For her own Good*. London: Pluto Press

Finch J & Groves D (eds) (1983) *A Labour of Love*. London: Routledge & Kegan Paul

Findley P (1939) *Priests of Luciria: The Story of Obstetrics*. Boston: Little, Brown & Co. (Quoted by Marieskind, p 286)

Grace Sister (1898) Practical aspects of nurses' life. *The Hospital*, Jan 8th, 127

Gamanikow E *et al.* (eds) (1983) *The Public and the Private*. London: Heinemann Educational Books

Graham H & Oakley A (1982) Competing ideologies of reproduction: medical and maternal perspectives on pregnancy. In White *et al.* (eds) *The Changing Experience of Women*. Oxford: Martin Robertson, in association with the Open University, 309–336

Graham H (1983) Caring: a labour of love. In Finch J & Groves (eds) *A Labour of Love*. London: Routledge & Kegan Paul, 13–30

Grant L (1983) Peer Expectations about oustanding competences of men and women medical students. *Sociology of Health and Illness*, **5** (1), 42–61

Hart N (1982) Explaining health inequality between the sexes. *Radical Community Medicine*, **11/12**, 25–34

Jex-Blake E (1886) Medical Women. Edinburgh: Oliphant Anderson & Ferrier Source Book Press, (Quoted by Marieskind, p 285)

Jordanova L J (1980) Natural facts: a historical perspective on science and sexuality. In MacCormack C & Strathen M (eds) *Nature, Culture and Gender: A Critique*. Cambridge University Press, 42–69

Kramer H & Sprenger J (1968) *'Malleus Male Ficarium' The Hammer of Witches*. Hughe P (ed) London Folio Society (Quoted by Ehrenreich B & English D, p 32)

Leanne J & Leanne J R L (1982) Alleged psychogenic disorders in women – a possible manifestation of sexual prejudice. In Whitelegg *et al*. *The Changing Experience of Women*. Oxford: Martin Robertson/Open University, 297–308

Leeson J & Gray J (1978) *'Women – Women and Medicine*. London: Tavistock Publications

Levin L S (1981) Self care in health. *World Health Forum*, **2**, 177–184

Magg S C (1984) Made not born. *Nursing Times*, **80** (19 Sept), 31–34

MacCormack C P (1980) Nature, culture and gender: a critique. In MacCormack C P & Strathen M (eds) *Nature, Culture and Gender*. Cambridge University Press

Marieskind H I (1980) *Women in the Health System*. St Louis, MO: C V Mosby Co

McLauren A (1977) The early birth control movement: an example of medical self help. In Woodward J & Richards D (eds) *Health Care and Popular Medicine in 19th Century England*. London: Croom Helm

M P U Policy Statement (1982) Discrimination against women. *Medical World*, Jan/Feb, 15

Muff J (ed) (1982) *Socialisation, Sexism and Stereotyping. Womens Issues in Nursing*, St Louis, MO: C V Mosby Co

Navarro V (1975) Women in health care. *New England Journal of Medicine*, **292**, 398–402 (Quoted by Clarke J)

Navarro V (1975) The industrialisation of fetishism for the fetisihism of industrialisation: a critique of Ivan Illich. *International Journal of Health Services*, **5** (3), 351–371

O'Connor M A (1984) *Self Help Groups in Health*. Unpublished M A Dissertation, London University

Parker R (1980) *The State of Care*. The Richard M. Titmuss Memorial Lecture, 1979–1980

Preston Whyte M E *et al* (1983) Effect of a principal's gender on consultation patterns. *Journal of the Royal College of General Practitioners*, **33**, (255), 654–658

Reynolds B (1982) Sex dictates trainers' choice. *Medeconomics*, December, 69–70

Roberts H (1981) Male hegemony in family planning. In Roberts H (ed) *Women, Health and Reproduction* London: Routledge & Kegan Paul, 1–17

Rosaldo M (1974) Women, Culture and Society. In Rosaldo M & Lamphere L (eds) *Women, Culture and Society*. Stanford University Press

Salmon B L (Chairman) (1966) *Report of the Committee on Senior Nursing Staff Structure*. London: HMSO

Savage W & Tate P (1983) Medical students attitudes towards women: a sex linked variable? *Medical Education*, **17**, 159–164

Scully D (1980) *Men who Control Women's Health* Boston: Houghton, Mifflin Co

Smith D (1975) The statistics of mental illness: what they will not tell us about women and why. In *Women Look at Psychiatry*. Vancouver: Vancouver Press Gang, 73–119

Ungerson C (1983) Women and caring: Skills, Tasks and Taboos. In Gamanikow E *et al.* (eds) *The Public and the Private*. London: Heinemann Educational Books, 62–77

Whitelegg E et al (eds) (1982) *The Changing Experience of Women*. Oxford: Martin Robertson/Open University

Woodward J & Richards D (1977) *Health Care and Popular Medicine in 19th Century England*. London: Croom Helm

Women's National Commission Report (1984) *Women and the Health Service*. WNC

WHO (1983) Women as providers of health care. *WHO Chronicle*, **37** (4), 134–138

Chapter 2

MAKING SENSE OF FEMINIST CONTRIBUTIONS TO WOMEN'S HEALTH

Anne Williams

One of the ways in which I have experienced feminism is through my interest in women's health. Recently, this interest has prompted me to look yet again at a growing number of publications written by women who are committed to exploring what it means to be a woman alive and healthy in the world today. These publications are sometimes referred to as being part of a feminist renaissance associated with works such as Betty Frieden's *Feminine Mystique*, Sheila Rowbotham's *Woman's Consciousness, Man's World*, and Ann Oakley's *Sex, Gender and Society*. Like earlier feminist writing, this literature is political and, as Liz Stanley writing in 1984 suggests, it argues from a position of involvement and passionate commitment.

For some, the passionate echoes in the word feminist can prove to be an obstacle to reading and understanding what is being said. However, as Janet Radcliffe Richards observes in her book *The Sceptical Feminist*, there is a danger that 'resistance to the feminist movement easily turns into a resistance to seeing that women have any problems at all' (Radcliffe Richards 1980, p 15). The problem contained within this statement has, it seems to me, special relevance for that part of the literature concerned with women's health. To ignore what is being written simply because it is labelled feminist may mean that I ignore, to my cost, information that has consequences for how I think about and act on health issues.

How, then, can this literature be approached? In this chapter, I try to read a number of published works in two ways. Firstly, as a critique of traditional views about women and health offered in, for example, medical textbooks and journals. Secondly, I shall also be attending to them as statements about feminism: that is to say, as affirmations of the hopes, ideas and intentions of women who contribute to the critique. This seems to me to be a useful approach which allows me to reject or accept what is written not simply because it bears the label 'feminist', but because it makes sense to me as a woman.

An early and landmark example of feminist health publications was the Boston Women's Health Collective's *Our Bodies, Ourselves* which was edited for use by women in Britain by Angela Phillips and Jill Rakusen. As the authors point out, the history of the book is long and satisfying. It began in 1969 with a small discussion group called Women and their Bodies, at a Boston Women's Conference. For most of the participants, talking amongst themselves about health issues was a totally new experience, and they decided to go on meeting as a group.

Part of their discussion turned on what they had learned about themselves in science or biology classes and books, and how what they had learned fell short of being relevant to their experiences. It also included expressing their feelings about medicine in general:

> 'We had all experienced frustration and anger towards specific doctors and the medical maze in general, and initially we wanted to do something about this.'
> (Phillips & Rakusen 1969, p 11)

Doing something involved further talk which led to the first inexpensive edition:

> 'As we talked we began to realize how little we knew about our bodies, so we decided to do further research, to prepare papers in groups and then to discuss our findings together. We learned from both professional sources (medical textbooks, journals, doctors, nurses) and from our own experience.'
> (Phillips & Rakusen 1969, p 11)

Learning from women's own experiences became central to the collective's efforts:

> 'The results of our findings were used to present courses for women. We would meet in any available free space, in schools, nurseries, church halls, in our own homes. As we taught, we learned from other women, and as they

learned, they went on to give courses to others. We saw it as a never-ending process always involving more and more women.'

(Phillips & Rakusen 1969, p 11)

The 'never ending process' has endured into the eighties, carrying in its wake an increasing number of publications. These vary in form from popular handbooks such as *The New Woman's Survival Catalog* (K Grimstad & S. Rennie 1973), and *New Woman's Health Handbook* (N McKeith 1978) to detailed essays such as 'Natural Facts' (L J Jordanova 1980) and collections of essays such as *Women, Health and Reproduction* (Helen Roberts 1981). Content ranges from specific health concerns, for example, alcoholism (eg. Brigid McConville 1983), smoking (eg. B Jacobson 1981), and compulsive eating (eg. Susie Orbach 1980), to discussion of social issues which impinge on women's life and health. Recent examples of this latter aspect include Janet Finch and Dulcie Groves' *A Labour of Love: Women, Work and Caring* (1983), and Hilary Graham's *Women, Health and the Family* (1984). One crucial and uniting factor is that all publications claim to discuss women's health issues within a feminist framework. When this claim to feminism is more closely examined, it seems to mean this: that while tone and opinion may differ, the writers are concerned with the gap between conventional views of health, offered in traditional medical and scientific writings, and their own and other women's everyday life experiences of what it feels like and means to be a healthy woman. This concern shines through the literature, whatever its emphasis, to illuminate at least two important features. These are, firstly, a move to redefine woman's health, basing definitions on the experiences of women, and secondly, a move to give women more control over their lives and over decisions that are made affecting their health.

Redefining women's health

A careful reading of the literature suggests that redefining women's health is at least a two-part process. The first part of the process is to look at how conventional arguments and views under criticism have been developed. The second part of the process involves constructing acceptable ways of thinking about women's health, that is to say, ways acceptable to women.

Criticising conventional views of women's health

Looking critically at how conventional medical views about women and health have been developed may have been implicit in early feminist writing, but on the whole the approach taken was to state that the medical view about matters such as contraception and childbirth was mistaken and oppressive, and to reject it. Only recently have serious analyses of these oppressive views been made. Lesley Doyal, writing in 1981, points to stark examples of conventional views of women's health, explaining that following Freud and despite the findings of Kinsey and Masters & Johnson, most doctors assume a neurotic basis for many of the problems presented by female patients. She continues:

> 'The medical belief in the inferiority of women is perhaps most clearly reflected in the widespread assumption that most women are basically 'neurotic'. This reflects much earlier ideas about the inherent sensitivity and irritability of women – ideas which have been reformulated in the light of recent developments in psychological and psychoanalytic theory.'
>
> (Doyal 1981, p 225)

L J Jordanova's analysis of these early ideas about women (1980) is interesting and perceptive. The view that women are highly sensible, meaning that they feel more acutely than men, was imaginatively built on during the enlightenment, Jordanova argues, to construct a whole image of the dependent nature of women. She goes on to show that these characteristics attributed to women by men served as the basis of a view that saw women as both passionate, ignorant, and inconsistent on the one hand, yet soft, moral, and civilising on the other. Overall, women were viewed as reactionary whereas men were seen as progressive. This view became so rigid that by the nineteenth century Michelet, a French writer, felt able to suggest that perhaps women were not responsible from a legal point of view in the same way that men were. Earlier, as Jordanova points out, William Cadogan, in his essay on nursing (1748), argued that 'the preservation of children should become the care of 'men of sense' because this business has been too long fatally left to the management of women'. Jordanova continues to discuss Cadogan:

'He justified the charge of female irresponsibility by invoking the 'superstitious practices and ceremonies' which they had inherited from 'their great grandmothers' . . . He recommended a transfer from female to male authority regarding infant care. He was not simply co-opting a new field for male medical practitioners for he also wished fathers to take a more active role . . . He never suggested that men take over the care of children, but that women should perform their alloted tasks under the advice of men, both their husbands and their doctors.'

(Jordanova 1980, p 51)

These ideas, which were constructed by an élite group of savants or intellectuals, bore no relationship to the messiness of the lived experience of the majority of the population. Rather were they constructed and exploited to advance these intellectuals; they were presented as knowledge to support a vision of science and medicine as the motors of social advance. Women, as Jordanova explains, 'occupied a peculiar position in the march of progress'. She then writes:

'On the one hand, their traditionalism had to be fought to the death, but, on the other hand, they had a major role to play in putting the family on a secure moral footing which was a necessary step in improving social life.'

(Jordanova 1981, p 65)

Analyses of this type are part of a wider study of the history of ideas, and since they are written from the standpoint of the present they can give insights into views held by their authors. So feminist analyses not only help us to understand the historical antecedents of women's oppression, they also speak about feminism. Jordanova's analysis is dense and thoughtful. One of its resounding echoes is how élite experience differs from everyday experiences of the rest of the population. But this idea is not presented as a simple dichotomy between, for example, oppressor and oppressed, rather understanding is sought through exploring 'contradictions, opposition, tensions and paradoxes' (Jordanova 1980, p 45).

An approach which takes everyday contradictions into

account provides useful insights into understanding women and health issues. Take the contradictions involved in being a woman and a doctor, as expressed by Gail Young (1981) in the following account:

> 'So in our culture, being a doctor inevitably involves conflict for a woman. There are practical conflicts with regard to home life and child rearing, conflicts about being female in a male sub-culture, conflicts about society's expectations and about her own self-expression. Whatever compromise she chooses, she will have difficulty in synthesising her self-image as a woman with her self-image as a doctor . . . Some people might say that the logical conclusion of all this is that women should not be doctors.'

She continues:

> 'I would counter that the doctor's role should change to allow people to be women in it. This means searching for ourselves our femaleness beyond the confines of the traditional role, and as we find ourselves, also finding ways of expressing ourselves at work. As a result medicine itself will change, become more female, more wholly human.'
> (Young 1981, p 156)

This example speaks of contradictions related to women and work and, more specifically, to issues associated with providing a context for health care. Contradictions, of course, pervade all health issues for women. The following example is taken from a conversation with a friend:

> 'I could not identify with the women's movement at the time of the abortion campaign because there was a conflict with my religion: a clash with my religious principles. As time had passed, I have looked at other feminist issues. For example, feminism has enlarged my view of God. The image of God as a man is limiting. If God has a gender, God is as much man as woman. I am a feminist but, for me, abortion is wrong. Speaking from the standpoint of not being pregnant or raped, abortion is murder in all instances.'*

---

* This is how I recorded part of a conversation I had with Tricia Black, a friend in October 1984.

To ignore contradictions in the lives of women is related to failing to take women seriously. Doyal underlines the importance of taking women seriously within health-related contexts. She comments that 'women have frequently described the reluctance of doctors to take seriously what they (the doctors) describe as minor ailments' (Doyal 1981, p 225). Amongst her examples are nausea and pain.

> 'Nausea . . . is experienced by over three-quarters of pregnant women. Each has a clearly identifiable physical cause. In childbirth, for example, pain is produced by strong contractions against a physical obstruction. Finally, symptom relief can be obtained relatively easily IF the problem is taken seriously. But despite such evidence, the medical belief in psychogenesis as the root of "female problems" remains extraordinarily persistent. Moreover, problems associated with female reproductive functioning are often attributed (at least implicitly) to the refusal of the woman in question to accept her 'femininity' at particular stages in her life. In the case of primary dysmenorrhea, for example, the adolescent girl is often said to be neurotic, with the implied cause being her incapacity to accept the onset of womanhood.'
>
> (Doyal 1981, p 226)

Constructing acceptable ways of viewing women's health

As feminist writers suggest, taking women seriously into account is not evident in conventional accounts of women and health. Any redefinition of women's health must take women and the contradictions of their lives seriously. This is asserted in feminist writing which relies on the messy, paradoxical, lived experiences of women to give substance to whatever the particular emphasis might be.

By way of example, let's look at pregnancy. Ann Oakley, in her book *From Here to Maternity: Becoming a Mother*, provides edited transcripts of women's experiences of what it means to become a mother. In her first chapter, she recounts the ways in which women first learn of their pregnancy, pointing out that often 'the body's response to conception may present a confused message, particularly for those women who were not planning a pregnancy' (Oakley 1981, p 29). Next, Oakley shows how women may feel about being pregnant. She suggests that at the beginning of pregnancy women may have mixed feelings. In her study, more than a third experienced this. The following account is illustrative:

> 'The first thing I did was cried. I was happy, but I was disappointed if you know what I mean. I was happy because when I wasn't getting pregnant I thought maybe there's something the matter with me . . . Then when I did get pregnant, I knew there was nothing wrong, and then I was disappointed to think I would have to give up my work, dear, because I had a very good job, I earned very good money.'
>
> (Oakley 1981, p 37)

And when the baby arrives? The following comments are extracts from responses to Oakley's question: 'Can you describe your feelings when you first held the baby?'

> 'Well, everyone says it's the most wonderful feeling, but I didn't feel, I felt pleased and everything, but not as much as I thought I would have done . . . I didn't really feel anything for her, not really, I thought it wasn't natural to feel like that, I thought then I didn't have a maternal instinct.'

And:

> 'I was very pleased. But I was very tired . . . afterwards and apart from feeling happy and pleased with myself that I had a lovely baby and it was a boy and everything else – I mean I didn't feel quite soppy, or anything, I wasn't really interested. In fact I was a bit worried that I wasn't interested. I thought I've got postnatal depression immediately!'
>
> (Oakley 1981, p 115–116)

In a later publication Oakley, with Hilary Graham (Graham & Oakley 1981, p 50–74), goes on to assert that views such as these contrast markedly with those of obstetricians. They write:

> 'Specifically, our data suggest that mothers and doctors disagree on whether pregnancy is a natural or a medical process and whether, as a consequence, pregnancy should be abstracted from the woman's life experience and treated as an isolated medical event.'
>
> (Graham & Oakley 1981, p 52)

They underline feminist thinking in stating that understanding pregnancy as an aspect of a woman's healthy life is tied-up and intimately enmeshed with other aspects of her life. Any redefinition of women's health cannot overlook this and, like conventional models, depend solely and simplistically on morbidity and mortality statistics. Referring to Kitzinger's work they emphasize how 'Because of the holistic way in which women view childbearing, the notion of successful reproduction is considerably . . . complex' (Graham & Oakley 1981, p 55). Refusal to consider and to be guided by women's experiences is to diminish understanding of women's health issues.

Thinking about women and health, using the experiences of women as a reference point, raises questions about interesting contingent issues such as women/health worker communication and the notion of 'professionals' as experts. What are the dimensions of the relationship between women and health care workers? Who are the experts? These questions prompt me, by way of exploration, to discuss what I consider to be a second interesting feature of the feminist literature, one that relates to the degree of control women have in their health care.

Taking control

In order to highlight this feature of the literature, I have found it useful to think about it in two ways. Firstly, to think about how women might gain more control over their health and wellbeing in their personal lives and, secondly, to consider what happens when women combine efforts and share experiences.

Personal control

Most feminists who write, particularly in the handbooks, talk about 'rediscovering ourselves as women' and 'valuing ourselves'. They stress the importance of knowledge in these processes. For example, to return to the Boston Women's Co-operative:

> 'Knowledge has freed us to an extent. It has freed us, for example, from playing the role of mother if it is not a role that fits us. It has given us room to discover the energy and talents that are in us.'
>
> (Phillips & Rakusen 1969, p 12–13)

What are the dimensions of this knowledge? What seems to persist through the literature, sometimes explicitly and often implicitly, is this: even biological facts appear in some kind of context, and 'facts' about women's anatomy and physiology can never be neutral. Even apparently sterile medical textbooks are not exempt, although they tend to be presented as 'correct'. Further and importantly, the feminist literature suggests that when anatomical and physiological facts are explored by women within the context of their feelings about their bodies and the meanings attached to bodily functions, the emerging knowledge is very different from that of the conventional literature: different in the sense that it is knowledge FOR women, not knowledge ABOUT women. The following quotation is apposite:

> 'Mothers view themselves as knowledgeable about pregnancy and birth. This knowledge stems not primarily from medical science, but rather from a woman's capacity to sense and respond to the sensations of her body. Rather than being an abstract knowledge acquired through formal training, it is thus an individualised and to some extent intuitive knowledge built up from bodily experiences (Boyle 1975; Goldthorpe & Richman 1976; McKinlay 1973).
> as quoted in (Graham & Oakley 1981, p 55)

An example of this kind of knowledge, where a woman knows what feels right or appropriate, is contained in dialogue offered by Graham & Oakley (1981) to illustrate conflicts in doctors' and pregnant mothers' frames of rererence for care:

Patient: I'm a hairdresser. I only do three days a week – is it all right to go on working?
Doctor: Up to twenty-eight weeks is all right on the whole, especially if you have a trouble-free pregnancy as you obviously have. After that its better to give up.
Patient: I only work three days a week, I feel fine.
Doctor: Yes, everything IS fine; but now you've got to this stage its better to give up, just in case.
(Graham & Oakley 1981, p 57)

The pregnant mother's feeling and knowledge of the situation is that she feels fine, but it is not taken seriously. The doctor's inclination, because of medical training, is to approach the situation as if things were or could be abnormal. She seems to be claiming that it does not matter how the pregnant woman feels, it is safer to go by the book.

Often, though, responding to feelings and knowing one's self is complicated by the impact of the views and ideas of the society in which one lives. It is all very well to be sure in the knowledge that one feels good or something feels right. What if knowing about oneself involves negative destructive feelings? Brigid McConville in *Women Under the Influence: Alcohol and Its Impact* (1983) describes aspects of the lives of a number of women who have come through severe drinking problems. To begin with, as McConville explains, each of the women 'felt that her problem – whether it had to do with sexuality, home, work, or marriage – was exclusively her own and in some way her own fault'. And:

> 'The guilt, anxiety and shame that each one felt, to be intensified in the vicious circle of dependent drinking, was in part a consequence of this sense of individual responsibility for "failure".'

However, she continues:

> 'In time, they each came to see their "failure" in terms of imposed social expectations about what women are supposed to be. Having once felt "wrong" for being "unable" to measure up to the stereotypical image of womanhood, they began to question whether there isn't something "wrong" with that image. In the process, they emerged from isolation, ceased to accept total blame for their drinking and came to see it in a wider context . . . '
>
> (McConville 1983, p 29)

Seeing or understanding things within a wider context is underlined by Susie Orbach, writing about compulsive eating:

> 'Underlying problems need to be exposed and separated though not necessarily worked through. The perspective is always to see the social dimensions that have led women to choose compulsive eating as an adaptation to sexist pressure in comtemporary society.'
>
> (Orbach 1978, p 14)

Here, knowledge is still based on feelings mediated by the experiences of living in the world, but things have come to be known in a different way. This, as several feminist publications show, can be liberating and allows for personal control over situations. A poignant example is taken from Jacobson's book *The Ladykillers*, where she talks about a woman who, while knowing that she was dying 'of smoking', was able to talk about why she was dying and to feel that she had at last some control over her life.

Women together

It is useful to note that accounts such as those I have just described are powerful: their publication affects and helps others. Part of the paradox of taking control of life and health is that the process, while personally important, is necessarily social. It involves sharing experiences. A feature of feminist contributions to health care is that they emphasise the importance of publishing the health experiences of women or sharing experiences through, for example, forming groups which provide a forum for support. Inevitably, these moves, by bringing women closer to each other, also have a powerful potential for changing existing relationships between women and institutions to give women greater control in the public arena. For example, women together have been effective in changing legislation and increasing access to having a greater say and choice over issues such as birth-control and abortion.

A key concept within this historical process of women gaining greater control over their health is the concept of 'rights'. Feminist literature is scattered with references to women's 'rights'. This raises in my mind some difficulties. For example, take the following statement:

> 'We know that a number of women and men believe sincerely that abortion is wrong. We cannot agree with them that an unborn fetus has more rights than a pregnant woman who is carrying it.'
> (Phillips & Rakusen 1978, p 293)

If I differentiate between rights, on what grounds do I do this? Take another example, the issue of pornography. A person may agree that material depicting women as objects of perverted sexual desire is inappropriate in public places, but they nevertheless often defend their right to use the material in private. For many, the material is demeaning in the very fact that it is produced, that it exists; others argue that, in certain places it cannot hurt but, as women who have come across such material and who have thought about the matter will agree, it still affects women by demeaning them, both individually and as a group.

Both abortion and sexual fulfilment, or lack of fulfilment, affect the health and well being of women. And it seems clear that both these issues of abortion and pornography raise difficulties concerning rights. For example, how do we balance the rights of the mother against the rights of the fetus, and the rights to behave freely in private against the rights of women not to be demeaned.

Recent feminist literature reflects, mainly implicitly, an awareness of these kinds of difficulties by recognising that while considerable advances have been made on issues of women's health on the 'rights' ticket, these advances are limited. For example, to say in 1975 that a change in the law would give women, not doctors, the right to choose in the case of abortion is only part of the battle. Implementation of rights does not take place in a social void but in the context, here, of relationships between health care workers and women. Professionals have power. As the literature I have discussed recognises, understanding this makes a difference, as well as being aware of rights and health care options. This is because women have experienced vulnerability in relationships with health professionals. Katy Gardner (1981) discusses the relationship between women and their doctors, and hints that doctors' power relates to their disease orientation and suggests that this means that they either 'medicalise' or 'trivialise' problems such as 'vaginal discharges, period pains, menopausal problems, cystitis', all of which she points out 'are far more relevant to women's everyday lives than "disease" as taught by hospitals' (Gardner 1981, p 131). To medicalise and trivialise diminishes that which women take seriously and does not provide women with what it is they want and need.

What clearly is called for is a change in the relationship between women and health professionals. What might this mean? Gardner provides some insights in what she has to say about well woman clinics. She looks at why women are the main consumers of health care. Her suggestions are:

'1 at present we assume the main responsibility for contraception;
2 women encounter the medical profession during pregnancy and childbirth;
3 we still assume prime responsibility for well and sick children;
4 women's anatomy seems more complex than men's and more likely to involve us in health problems and illness;
5 traditionally women have been seen as frail and doctors have capitalised on women's weaknesses by inventing treatments, for the "vapours", etc. Although the day of the vapours has gone, women still see themselves as ill more often than men – men who are distressed may go to the pub – women go to the doctor.'

(Gardner 1981, p 130–131)

Looking at this list, two things present themselves as being particularly interesting. Firstly, women consult doctors not so much about their own health but about problems relating to responsibilities they have undertaken such as contraception, looking after children, and caring for other dependents; that is, it is as carers for others that they are prime users of the health service. The following question is raised: to what extent is medical *advice* appropriate, or is it *support* that is needed for women in this role as society's carers? Secondly, there is the point about women seeing themselves as ill, which of course relates to the claim that women's lives have been medicalised (see Illich 1979). This is a feature of the history of women and their health of which feminist writers are well aware. Katy Gardner does not see well woman clinics as an attempt further to medicalise women's lives, but rather as an attempt to provide an open access system where any woman can go to have a check-up and discuss matters which concern them about their health and well-being with health care workers. Support, discussion and open access are key words in attempts to try to alter the relationship between women and health professionals. Gardner's discussion of the Islington Clinic documents, the part played by a well woman clinic in this respect (Gardner 1981, p 129–143), as do accounts elsewhere, for example in other chapters in this volume, where the emphasis is on supportive, participative care.

Summary

I have outlined what I consider to be crucial features of a number of feminist publications which, although varied in emphasis and tone, put forward a view of women and health which calls into question orthodoxies which have long influenced health professionals and policy-makers.

The first feature is a redefinition of women's health. This I have suggested is a two-part process which involves critical examination of conventional medical views and, following this, the construction of views of health which take into account the experiences of women. What strikes me about this feature is recognition on the part of most feminist authors of the complexities involved in writing about women's health and an insistence on underlining the contradictions so often experienced by women and which orthodox medical texts obscure or ignore entirely.

The second feature common to feminist publications is a demand that women be enabled to gain much greater control over their bodies, health and lives. Typical ways in which greater control can be achieved include, notably, increased awareness of health matters among women and, particularly, awareness of the sorts of contradictions described here. Further, feminist writers encourage me to take the everyday puzzles in my life seriously enough to share them with other women and to explore, with other women, experiences which question stereotypical images of women.

All this seems to me to mean change; change through transforming personal experience into a political commitment to working towards healthier lives for women. Within the publications I have referred to, I can find no hard and fast answers, no neat packages to help me. What I do find is affirmation of my own feelings about what it means to be a healthy woman alive in today's world, and the encouragement to participate in advancing those changes which I find make sense to me as a woman.

References

Doyal L (1980) *The Political Economy of Health*. London: Pluto Press

Finch J & Groves D (eds) (1983) *A Labour of Love: Women, Work and Caring*. London: Routledge & Kegan Paul

Friedan B (1963) *The Feminine Mystique*. Harmondsworth: Penguin Books

Gardner K (1981) Well woman clinics. In Roberts H (ed) *Women, Health and Reproduction*. London: Routledge & Kegan Paul.

Graham H (1984) *Women, Health, and the Family*. Brighton, Sx: Wheatsheaf Books

Graham H & Oakley A (1981) Medical and maternal perspectives on pregnancy. In Roberts H (ed) *Women, Health and Reproduction*. London: Routledge & Kegan Paul

Grimstad K Rennie S (1973) *The New Woman's Survival Catalog*. New York: Coward, McCann & Geoghegan

Illich I (1979) *Limits to Medicine*. Harmondsworth: Penguin Books

Jacobson B (1981) *The Ladykillers: Why smoking is a Feminist Issue*. London: Pluto Press

Jordanova L J (1980) Natural facts. In MacCormack C & Strathern M (eds) *Nature, Culture and Gender*. Cambridge University Press

McConville B (1983) *Women Under the Influence*. London: Virago Press

McKeith N (1978) *The New Women's Health Handbook*. London: Virago Press

Oakley A (1972) *Sex, Gender and Society*. London; Temple Smith

Oakley A (1979) *From Here to Maternity*. Harmondsworth: Penguin Books

Oakley A Mitchell J (1976) *The Rights and Wrongs of Women*. Harmondsworth: Penguin Books

Orbach S (1980) *Fat is a Feminist Issue*. London: Hamlyn Paperbacks

Phillips A Rakusen J (1969) *Our Bodies, Ourselves*. Harmondsworth: Penguin Books

Radcliffe Richards J (1980) *The Sceptical Feminist*. Harmondsworth: Penguin Books

Roberts H (ed) (1981) *Women, Health and Reproduction*. London: Routledge & Kegan Paul

Rowbotham S (1973) *Woman's Consciousness; Man's World*. Harmondsworth: Penguin Books

Stanley Liz (1984) Why men oppress women. In Webb S & Pearson C (eds) *Looking Back in Studies in Sexual Politics No. 1*. Department of Sociology, Manchester University

Young G (1981) A Woman in medicine: reflections from the inside. In Roberts H (ed) *Women, Health and Reproduction*. London: Routledge & Kegan Paul

Chapter 3

DEFINING WOMEN AND THEIR HEALTH – THE CASE OF HYSTERECTOMY

Christine Webb

Gender stereotyping has gone on from the beginning of recorded history, and women have been defined by men as inferior to themselves and suited to a particular range of social activities as a result of their different reproductive functions. In this chapter, we shall trace some of these trends as they have related to women both as givers and receivers of health care, and shall see how in the last century psychological theories have come to the fore and have been used to define women when they are healthy and when they are sick. The particular example of hysterectomy will be discussed to illustrate this process of categorising women as ruled by their psychology and their emotions.

We live in a patriarchal – or male-dominated – society, and the evidence of its effects on women's lives is everywhere around us. Even in a profession like nursing, where the majority of nurses are women, top-level posts are increasingly held by men (Nuttall 1983; Pollock & West 1984). The same happens in teaching and in infant schools, in particular, women make up the majority of teachers but men occupy a disproportionate number of head teacher positions. In medicine, the general pattern is the same but is complicated by the hierarchy of prestige attaching to different specialities. There are not only few women professors and deans of medical schools, but men predominate in surgery, neurology, cardiology and other high status areas, while women are to be found concentrated in general practice, in jobs which link with traditional definitions of 'women's work' such as paediatrics, and in areas where part-time work is easier and so can be fitted in with childcare responsibilities (Oakley 1981).

The origins of this male power structure have been traced to biological, psychological and social influences, but whether hormones, the nervous system, needs, drives, instincts or socialisation are *the* determinant seems irrelevant at this stage in our social development. It is probably more useful to devote energy to wiping out systematic discrimination based on gender, for the fact that women and men are anatomically different does not mean that one is better than the other. To rank one as inferior and the other as superior is to make a value judgement which is unscientific, immoral and just plain wasteful of people's talents – both women and men.

Wherever sex stereotypes originated, they are certainly well-established now, and are socially transmitted by ideologies and social practices. 'Scientific' theories have been used throughout history to justify male domination in society in general and in medicine in particular. Feminist historians, however, have recently shown how important women's contribution to health care has been in the past. Women have always been the largest numbers of health care workers, just as they are today, and have always treated people both in professional, paid occupations and as lay carers in their own and other people's homes (Mitchell & Oakley 1976; Ehrenreich & English 1979). High and low social class women have practised health care even when they were excluded by men of the Church or State from studying medicine formally or from gaining an official licence to practice.

Women carers in the community in the Middle Ages are often described as witches, and a new 'myth' has built up that thousands of them were persecuted and put to death. It is certainly true that women were effective carers on a wide scale, and that their remedies were based on long experience with herbs and other types of remedies. They learned their skills from their mothers or other women, and assisted at normal and abnormal births, probably carried out abortions for women desperate in the face of repeated pregnancies, and disposed of deformed or unwanted babies. The doctors of the time, by contrast, based their practice not on empirical evidence but on abstract, religious theories of humours, vapours, and dispositions. However, there were very few doctors and they confined their practice to towns where the most lucrative opportunities were available, and women working in rural areas and poorer urban areas were thus no real threat to them. Therefore, it is likely that the extent of persecution of women witches has been exaggerated (Hasted 1984).

Nevertheless, it is accurate to say that women have always constituted the majority of both professional and lay health workers, and that 'old wives' tales' were the fruit of an apprenticeship with an older and more experienced woman who passed on her accumulated wisdom to the next generation. More scientific medicine began in the 18th century, according to Foucault, with the opening of the body to the 'gaze'. With the acceptance by the Church of dissection, doctors could actually look in to bodies to study disease processes and 'the living night was dissipated in the brightness of death' (Foucault 1973). This development meant that doctors needed 'material' for study and they turned for this to hospitals for the lower social classes. In the USA, for example, Sims – who invented the speculum – kept a group of black women slaves in a compound and experimented on them to develop his gynaecological surgery techniques, particularly repair of vesicovaginal fistulae. He operated on one woman over 30 times in four years, but repeated infections led to failure each time. The women were given opium as an analgesic and this perpetuated their dependence both on the drug and on Sims who supplied it. Later he moved to New York and continued experimenting on poor Irishwomen in the wards of New York Women's Hospital (Ehrenreich & English 1979).

While the poor suffered from medical experimentation, upper class women suffered from doctor's medical practice. In the 19th century, a 'mysterious epidemic' seemed to attack middle and upper-class women (Ehrenreich & English 1979). The condition was variously labelled neurasthenia, nervous prostration and hysteria, and the symptoms were those of general debility. Women became pale and thin, and were too weak to engage in any activities except lying on a sofa or bed. Famous sufferers from this state include Florence Nightingale herself, and Harriet Martineau, a political economist. Poor women did not suffer from the condition, and some feminists of the time – including Olive Schreiner and Charlotte Perkins Gilman – saw the link between female illness and upper-class women's economic and social situation. They had no serious work to do, for servants did the housework and looked after the children. The only functions of the upper class woman were sexual and reproductive, and beyond this she was merely an article of conspicuous consumption which demonstrated the financial success of her husband. It is easy to see the similarities between 19th-century problems of this nature and the depression experiences by isolated women housewives today (Hobson 1978).

As well as being restricted in their roles, 19th-century women were literally physically restricted in their movements by tight corsets and heavy clothing which led in the short-term to shortness of breath, constipation, weakness and indigestion and in the long-term to bent or fractured ribs, displacement of the liver and uterine prolapse or even procidentia. This may be equated with the Chinese practice of footbinding and Ehrenreich & English (1979) call it 'paternalistic necrophilia', because men of the time were apparently attracted to women disabled and crippled in this way.

Doctors developed the theory that woman's normal state was to be sick, because female functions were inherently pathological. This particularly applied to her monthly periods, which were seen as a sickness which necessitated rest and suspension of any physical activity such as long walks, dancing, riding and socialising. A pregnant woman was thought to be indisposed throughout the pregnancy, which was therefore called a 'confinement', and when her childbearing years ended she entered the menopause, or phase of terminal illness. Working-class women were not considered to be susceptible to these problems, because they were physically more robust and did not suffer from the same sensitivities as more 'refined' women.

Some doctors of the time believed that the uterus was the controlling female organ, but others attributed this role to the ovary and developed a whole 'psychology of the ovary'. Those adhering to the 'uterus' version believed that 'hysteria' was due to a 'wandering womb', and they prescribed concoctions to be inserted into the vagina either to attract the uterus back into its place or cause it to move to a more auspicious position. These substances varied from tea and marshmallow to leeches. Education for women was not advised because it supposedly led to masculinisation, difficulty in breast feeding, or even disappearance of the breasts. Too much reading could cause permanent damage to the reproductive organs, and women should rest a great deal to focus energy downwards to the uterus and regulate their periods. Higher education could even cause uterine atrophy and medical training for women was, of course, particularly prejudicial to their health.

Apart from instillations into the vagina and removal of the ovaries, the rest cure was popular among doctors in the 19th century. This consisted of long periods of total isolation and sensory deprivation, soft foods and massages. But above all, the cure depended on the doctor-patient relationship, which demanded absolute submission and obedience to the doctor's control. Female doctors would obviously be quite unsuitable for such work.

With the discovery of hormones in the 1920s, the uterus-brain link became the focus of medical attention and gynaecologists ventured more and more into management of the 'total patient', aided by Freudian theory which began to spread in the same period. According to Freud, little girls become aware at about the age of three or four that they have no penis, and they feel castrated as a result. They blame their mothers for this and suffer from penis envy for the rest of their lives. Girls' childhood sexuality is said to be centred on the clitoris, but with increasing maturity sexuality should be transferred to the vagina and women who fail to do this are thus immature. Those who do not accept their maturity, natural femininity and sexuality by having children are denying themselves the masochistic satisfaction of childbirth (Deutsch 1945). Female sexuality, for Freud, was essentially passive, matching the inactive, recipient role of the ovum in fertilisation, compared with the active, seeking role of the sperm.

Thus the whole of a woman's personality sprang from her reproductive functions, and psychological disorders developed from her failure to accept this rather than from her realisation that men have much greater opportunities to take up a range of activities and occupations. Freud claimed that women envied men their penises, when in reality women were envying the greater life chances from which they were excluded. Even when the fundamental tenets of Freudian theory in relation to female sexuality had been disproved (Kinsey *et al.* 1948; 1953; Masters & Johnson 1966), medical textbooks continued to be based on his ideas. Diane Scully and Pauline Bart, two American sociologists, examined 27 general gynaecology textbooks published in the USA between 1943 and 1973 to assess how far they reflected the findings of Kinsey, Masters and Johnson. They found that two-thirds of the books published between 1963 and 1972, the period immediately following important discoveries by sexuality researchers, failed to discuss the issue of the clitoral versus the vaginal orgasm. Eight books continued to state that the male sex drive was stronger, and half still maintained that procreation was the major function of sex for the female. Two repeated that the vaginal orgasm was the only mature response for a woman. Scully & Bart comment:

> 'Gynecologists, our society's official experts on women, think of themselves as the woman's friend; with friends like that, who needs enemies?'

Thus, women continue to be defined as appendages of their genital organs, with personalities which are inherently less active, ambitious, rational and intellectual than those of men. While gynaecologists still play an extensive role in this kind of social control of women by defining and treating them as inferior to and different from men, as we shall see when we discuss the example of hysterectomy, psychotherapy and psychotropic drugs have also become important agents for the social control of women. For example, despite the existence of acceptable evidence of their physiological origins, numerous 'women's problems' have been given a psychogenic label, including dysmenorrhoea, pain in labour, infant colic, and 'trivial' side-effects of contraceptive measures (Birke & Gardner 1979; Lennane & Lennane 1982).

Social control mechanisms now focus on the mind, or the soul as Foucault (1975) puts it, whereas previously they concentrated on the body. In patriarchal society, male domination is justified and transmitted ideologically, that is through ideas which are put forward as natural but which in reality are devices for manipulating and misleading people about the truth (Larrain 1979). We have seen that Freudian ideas have been very influential in the social control of women, and that they portray 'essential womanhood' as passive, emotional and lacking in ambition. The medical literature on hysterectomy is no exception, and in fact can be seen as the archetype of this view of women as ruled by their reproductive organs, either by direct psychological links or via the hormones.

Doctors' writings on hysterectomy

The main preoccupation of both gynaecologists and psychiatrists studying hysterectomy is 'poor outcome', defined as increased levels of depression after the operation. This depression is seen as a natural and inevitable result of damage to the 'feminine self-concept' because 'completeness as a woman' is lost (Raphael 1972). In the course of a study of recovery from hysterectomy, Webb & Wilson-Barnett (1983) reviewed over sixty articles in medical journals from a large number of different countries, and they found early psychoanalytic workers such as Helen Deutsch (1945) and Marvin Drellich & Irving Bieber (1958) quoted as fundamental sources in almost all of them. As with Scully & Bart's review of medical textbooks, the fact that Freudian ideas had been heavily criticised and in some instances shown to be false, seemed to have been ignored by writers on hysterectomy.

In Deutsch's *Some Psychoanalytic Observations in Surgery* (1942), she notes that her observations result, not from planned collection of data in a systematic way, but from long years of psychoanalytic experience. These observations show her that fear of castration is a specific fear related to surgery, that some patients perceive operations as punishments for masturbation, and that postoperative depression may be a sign of surrender to the 'punishing forces'. In female patients there is said to be 'an interplay between pregnancy and birth fantasies on the one hand and castration complex on the other'. The diseased organ, in addition, frequently has 'an extremely personified significance: it then becomes the most loved part of the whole body, a second, beloved little self'. Sometimes the organ is seen by patients to be a persecutor. Post-operative reactions are dependent on the woman's relationship to the organ concerned, but 'the castration complex stands in the centre of the anxieties'.

Drellich & Bieber's (1958) study of 23 premenopausal women undergoing hysterectomy for benign or malignant disease is typical of many later studies in not distinguishing between cancer and non-cancer surgery. By focusing on 'the psychological importance of the uterus and its functions' they imply that this is the main concern for women, rather than the fact that they may have a malignant condition. This assumption is explicitly made by Derogatis (1980), who says that 'the issue of sexuality is *central* rather than subordinate in their appreciation of the impact of cancer' (emphasis in the original). Patients in the Drellich & Bieber study had bilateral removal of the ovaries together with hysterectomy, but the authors do not point out that this invalidates their conclusions about the effect of a simple hysterectomy, because their patients simultaneously experienced a sudden onset of the menopause. Using the usual Freudian Catch 22, Drellich & Bieber state:

> 'It is easy to demonstrate that most women have a wish to bear and raise children. Furthermore, psychoanalysis of women who have no conscious wish for children often reveals pregnancy wishes which are disguised or repressed because of fears or inhibitions.'
> (Drellich & Bieber 1958)

Most of the women they studied expressed spontaneous regret over loss of their ability to become pregnant again, but some denied apprehension over the loss of their reproductive organs and 'some consciously seemed to welcome the operation, but this was often a denial of intolerable feelings of impending loss' in the researchers' interpretation. Two other women '*appeared* to welcome the operation because it eliminated the possibility of undesired pregnancy and would relieve them of the burden of previous troublesome contraceptive techniques' (my emphasis). Drellich & Bieber place less reliance on women's own explanations and seem to think that their phychoanalytic interpretation will be meaningful to the women themselves when they write:

> 'Attitudes expressed by a woman towards the uterus and its real or imagined functions should be regarded as specific expressions of her attitudes towards herself as a woman and her feminine role in life.'

They suggest that the psychoanalytic concept of castration is close to that encountered in males when their sexual organs are removed, and that recovery problems after hysterectomy are related to 'castration anxiety'. Menstruation is also said to be 'a necessary and valued function whose termination was viewed with regret', and compulsive eating may occur after hysterectomy as women attempt to fill the void created by loss of their 'internal penis'. Menzer *et al.* (1957) also consider that 'attitude towards femininity' is one of the most important factors in emotional adjustment of hysterectomy. Their phraseology is similar to that already discussed, as Polivy shows:

> 'Those who did well (after hysterectomy) either denied themselves feminine gratifications, turning instead to masculine occupations or pursuits, or resolved satisfactorily the loss of reproductive functioning. The patients who adjusted poorly were all married women with children whose 'masochism' had supposedly been incompletely gratified in the female reproductive functions.'
>
> (Polivy 1974)

This echoes Deutsch's proposal of a uterus-pregnancy-birth triad as a source of masochistic pleasure for women.

These themes recur throughout the more recent literature, and many doctors suggest that regrets or conflicts over loss of childbearing capacity lead to 'poor outcome' (Ackner 1960; Barglow *et al.* 1963; Steiner & Aleksandrowicz 1970). For example, Barglow *et al.* (1965) studied 72 pregnant 'patients' and allocated them randomly to either a tubal ligation or hysterectomy group. All these women 'had shown an interest in surgical sterility, though few had actively sought it' (Polivy 1974). More hysterectomy than tubal ligation patients subsequently had a 'poor response', which the authors attribute to the fact that hysterectomy is so final, whereas with tubal ligation women can maintain a fantasy that the tubes might come untied. Barglow considers that, as long as pregnancy is still even theoretically possible, women feel intact. He does not consider the possibility that the women's unhappiness might have had any connection with being subjected to an operation to which they did not freely consent. Other suggested causes of 'poor outcome' include neurotic personality, an addiction to surgery (Polivy 1974), psychiatric illness (Melody 1962; Barker 1968; Gath 1980), or 'functional' (ie. psychosomatic) disorders (Barker 1968; Richards 1973).

Patterson & Craig (1963) are highly critical of psychoanalytic interpretations of outcome from hysterectomy, both because of their methodology and their findings. They believe that the psychoanalytic interview is based on 'beliefs which stem from impressions and the latter are spawned by the colourful and captivating accounts of a few patients'. This convinces analysts of the correctness of their interpretations. Patterson & Craig used open-ended interview techniques to study post-hysterectomy patients and found that they did not consider themselves mutilated, were contented with sterilisation, and did not long for the masochistic pleasure of childbirth. This suggests to them that male concern about castration has led unjustifiably to the belief that women must think along the same lines. However, since the uterus and ovaries are not visible, while the male organs are external and are seen and handled several times each day, the female body picture is different from that of the male. Helen Deutsch's proposal of the necessity for women of masochistic pleasure in pregnancy and childbirth is criticised as a projection of her own thinking, and this idea received no support in Patterson & Craig's study. They conclude that 'these occasional romantic case histories do not justify generalisation'. The fact that Patterson & Craig's dissenting report has had relatively little influence on gynaecological and psychiatric writings about recovery from hysterectomy is an indication of how firmly established are psychoanalytic theories.

A study of recovery from hysterectomy

This literature formed the background to a study by Webb & Wilson-Barnett (1983) of recovery from hysterectomy, in which 128 women were interviewed in hospital and followed up four months later at home. We were interested in finding out what women themselves felt about having a hysterectomy and about their recovery, how they evaluated their own progress, and whether they were depressed during convalescence.

Two women nurse researchers carried out interviews using structured schedules comprised mainly of open-ended questions, and women were also asked to complete the Beck Depression Inventory (Beck *et al.* 1961) at the end of each interview. All the women interviewed had heard so-called 'old wives' tales', and were concerned that the operation might make them put on weight, age rapidly, grow facial hair, become depressed, lose interest in sex or be a less satisfying sexual partner. As a result, only 68% had actually wanted to have a hysterectomy, while 22% had definitely not wanted it. The remainder felt they had had no choice, either because of the severity of their heavy, painful and irregular menstrual bleeding with its accompanying distress, tiredness and irritability or because their doctor could offer no alternative effective treatment.

We asked women how they felt about losing their periods and fertility, and their replies are summarised in Table 3.1. This shows that the majority were happy to have no more periods, and they expressed this quite strongly in terms such as 'wonderful', 'marvellous' and 'I'm saving a fortune!' Those who did not know how they felt about this and about not being able to become pregnant again said it was too soon after the operation to be sure how they felt. With regard to loss of fertility, again many were very positive about their feelings, saying 'great' or 'it's a big relief'. The nine who were unhappy not to be able to become pregnant included three who had had unsuccessful investigations for infertility in the past and one who had been sterilised and then remarried. She had been sterilised immediately after her second child was born because her doctor had said it would be dangerous to have another child due to the fact that she had had a brain haemorrhage during pregnancy. She had immediately regretted being sterilised and felt her consent had not been valid because she had still been under the influence of drugs given to relieve pain during labour. Thus, all those with regrets had particular and unusual reasons for them.

Table 3.1 Women's opinions about losing the periods and fertility. (Figures are percentages and relate to the 103 women who were premenopausal before operation)

	Happy	Unhappy	Don't know	Total
How do you feel about not having any more periods?	94	1	5	100
How do you feel about not being able to become pregnant any more?	84	9	7	100

When we asked, 'Overall, how do you feel about having had a hysterectomy?', 89% gave 'positive' replies such 'I'm glad I had it – I should have done it years ago but I was afraid' and 'Good. It was the best day's work I ever did.' Similarly, almost all said they would advise another woman to have the operation if she needed it, and not to pay any attention to 'old wives' tales'. Nobody said she was sorry or regretted having the operation, but 11% were unsure whether having it had been a good thing or not. The same women expressed doubts when we asked a number of other questions such as 'Do you feel life has returned to normal after your operation?' and 'How is your health now compared with what it was like before?'

We analysed these women's experiences to try to discover why they were dissatisfied, and found that they had had one or more serious physical complications during convalescence. These were wound, vaginal and urinary infections which had been treated by antibiotics. Some women were now free of infection but their recovery was held up by tiredness as a result of the infection and its treatment. Others were still not cured of their infections and had to wear pads because of vaginal discharge associated with incomplete healing and infection, or still had cystitis with its accompanying frequency and burning on passing urine.

We used scores on the Beck Depression Inventory to measure levels of depression at both interviews, as well as asking women themselves if they had been depressed. At the first interview in hospital five days after operation, 121 of the 128 women had 'not depressed' scores, which suggests that hysterectomy patients are not a depressed group, and at the four-month follow-up interview 123 were 'not depressed'. Statistical comparisons of these scores over the study period showed that average depression levels had decreased over the study period ($p = 0.001$), which runs counter to suggestions by doctors that there are high levels of depression following hysterectomy.

We analysed all interview and Beck Depression Inventory data to check the effects of factors said in the medical literature to lead to 'poor outcome'. Again our findings contradicted medical reports in that no effect was found for age, number of children, desire for more children, marital status, menopausal status, psychiatric history, surgical history, medical history or personality.

Our overall impression from interviewing these 128 women was that they felt healthier, both physically and psychologically, did not regret losing their periods and fertility, and were glad they had had the operation. They had often delayed having a hysterectomy and had put up with distressing and debilitating pain and bleeding for months or even years, but now their own experiences led them to disbelieve the pessimistic 'old wives' tales' they had heard. By their own accounts and on Beck Depression Inventory scores, they were less depressed 4 months after their operation and they attributed this to relief of their physical symptoms.

Whose old tales?

The phrase 'old wives' tales' is widely used in a pejorative sense to suggest inaccurate, unscientific information based on ignorance and passed around by women, in contrast to empirically-validated, scientific male knowledge (Versluysen, 1980). Its effect is to devalue and trivialise women's knowledge, which in reality is usually based on the practice and experience of care, while male 'science' is often unverified theorising (Ehrenreich & English 1979). Other women's knowledge about hysterectomy passed on to women in our study was largely experience transmitted via oral accounts from earlier generations. It was very probably an accurate representation of the experiences of the women's forebears, but as such could not reflect more recent trends. Hysterectomy was undoubtedly an extremely traumatic physical and emotional event when the ovaries were routinely removed at the same time, and when women were kept in bed for weeks after operation, and consequently had a long struggle to regain their strength and health. 'Old wives' tales' were therefore accurate for the time they describe.

In contrast, 'scientific' reports in the medical literature reflect a systematic bias because they are based on psychoanalytic preconceptions about women's sexuality and psychology. In addition, their research methodology is dubious in numerous ways. As a result, they repeat ideological misrepresentations of women's experiences and thereby set the scene for self-fulfilling prophecies. Doctors expect women to react to hysterectomy by becoming depressed. They spread these ideas amongst themselves and communicate them to women, too. Because medical opinion appears to validate what women have heard about their mothers' and grandmothers' hysterectomies years earlier, it is hard for women's more recent experiences to replace out of date information. The phrase 'old doctors' tales' is an appropriate description of these medical misrepresentation, provided we remember that their truth-value is very different from that of 'old wives' tales'.

Towards a feminist approach to hysterectomy

This study raises important and complex issues for feminists. I suggest that doctors' focus on psychological problems during recovery reflects the influence of psychoanalytic ideology in medicine, with a consequent stereotyping of women as emotionally unstable and reacting to events in their lives by developing psychological disturbances. While the majority of women in the study were pleased to have had a hysterectomy, did not feel diminished and unfeminine, and did not become depressed, its adverse effects are significant. All women had undergone a painful and distressing operation followed by varying degrees of suffering during convalescence. Their family and social lives had been disrupted and they had been financially penalised by the extra expenses involved in being ill, as well as by inability to work for several months.

The problems of those whose recovery was not smooth pose a fundamental challenge to medical interpretations because these women had *physical* and not psychological complications. In all, over 50% of the women had been prescribed antibiotics at some stage in their recovery, either in hospital or at home. Some had had more than one course of treatment. Furthermore, these infections were potentially preventible, their causes lying in techniques of surgery and thus with doctors themselves (Richardson & Lyon 1981). Doctors seem to find it easier to attribute complications to women's psychology rather than to examine their own practice and remedy its defects.

Another telling finding of the study is that 28% of women had no abnormality of the uterus when it was examined in the laboratory after the operation. In some medical reports this incidence is even higher. During our literature search we came across no medical research into causes of irregular menstrual bleeding which might lead to making more refined diagnoses and devising less invasive treatments. Many women had had 'trials' of hormone tablets or a dilatation and curettage to see whether their bleeding could be controlled, but none had had investigations of their hormone levels. Nor did we come across any research looking into possible environmental, dietary or other influences on menstruation. I conclude, as others have done (Rugen unpublished), that 'women's troubles' are not considered important and interesting enough to merit the attention of medical scientists. This is a logical extension of their assumption that women's problems have psychological origins.

Clearly, feminists would not want to advocate hysterectomy as a quick and easy way of dealing with menstrual irregularities or support its almost routine use for women aged 35 or over as seems to be happening in the USA. Gynaecological surgery as currently practised is 'a socially sanctioned genital trauma performed by males on females' (Scully 1980) which is largely outside women's own control and decision-making, as shown by the numbers of women in the study who did not want the operation. But for some women whose lives are being made miserable by heavy, prolonged, irregular menstrual bleeding, hysterectomy may be the only solution available at the present. They need to have accurate information about the operation and its effects, how they will feel afterwards, and how various aspects of their lives may or may not be affected. Experience shows that this is unlikely to come from doctors, and so women must seek and provide it themselves. Some hysterectomy self-help groups have already been set up and well woman clinics may be a resource for this purpose. A contact address is given at the end of the chapter.

I feel that nurses, the majority of whom are women themselves, should play a special role in helping women with health problems and giving information to those deciding whether to have a hysterectomy, going through the experience in hospital and recovering at home afterwards. Unfortunately, women in our study did not get the kind of help they needed from nurses while in hospital and they were very critical of this aspect of their experience.

Research is also needed into all aspects of menstruation and, if this is to focus on aspects which are meaningful and relevant for women themselves, it is clear that they must be involved in deciding research objectives and methods, and using the findings. Some research, for example hormone studies, will need technical resources, but it is likely that environmental and life-style factors could be investigated by groups of women without a lot of equipment and funds. For example, an endometriosis self-help group has begun to computerise the history of members to try to find links between life-style, previous medical history, type of contraception used, and so on, and endometriosis.

Treatment of women having a hysterectomy takes place within a male- and medically-dominated health care system which stereotypes women as irrational, emotional and defined by their reproductive systems. These suggestions can therefore at best only help to make women's treatment a little more tolerable. They are plainly not a substitute for feminist analysis and collective action directed towards ending the systematic oppression of women by patriarchal institutions.

Useful addresses

Endometriosis Self-help Group, c/o Ailsa Irving, 65 Holmdene Avenue, London SE24 9LD

Hysterectomy Support Group, c/o Judy Vaughan, Rivendell, Warren Way, Lower Heswall, Wirral, Merseyside

Pelvic Inflammatory Disease Self-help Group c/o Jessica Pickard, 32 Parkholme Road, London E8

Women's Health Information Centre, 53 Featherstone Street, London EC1

References

Ackner B (1960) Emotional aspects of hysterectomy. In Jores A & Freyburger H (eds) *Advances in Psychosomatic Medicine*. New York: Karger

Barglow P, Gunther M S, Johnson A & Meltzer H J (1965) Hysterectomy and tubal ligation: a psychiatric comparison. *Obstetrics & Gynecology*, **25** (4), 520–527

Barker M G (1968) Psychiatric illness after hysterectomy. *British Medical Journal*, **2**, 91–95

Beck A T, Ward C H, Mendelson M Mock J & Erbaugh J (1961) An inventory for measuring depression. *Archives of General Psychiatry*, **4**, 561–571

Birke L & Gardner K (1979) *Why Suffer? Periods and their Problems*. London: Virago

Deutsch H (1942) Some psychoanalytic observations in surgery. *Psychosomatic Medicine*, **4**, 105–115

Deutsch H (1942) *The Psychology of Women*. New York: Grune & Stratton

Derogatis L R (1980) Breast and gynecological cancers: their unique impact on body image and sexual identity in women. In Vaeth J M (ed) *Frontiers of Radiation Therapy and Oncology*, **14** 1–11. Basel: Karger

Drellich M G & Bieber I (1958) The psychological importance of the uterus and its function: some psychoanalytic implications of hysterectomy. *Journal of Nervous and Mental Diseases*, **126**, 322–336

Ehrenreich B & English D (1979) *For her Own Good. 100 Years of the Experts' Advice to Women*. London: Pluto Press

Foucault M (1973) *The Birth of the Clinic*. London: Tavistock Publications

Foucault M (1977) *Discipline and Punish. The Birth of the Prison*. London: Allen Lane

Gath D (1980) Psychiatric aspects of hysterectomy. In Rubins L, Clayton P & Wing J (eds) *The Social Consequences of Psychiatric Illness*. New York: Brunner Mazel

Hasted R (1984) The new myth of the witch. *Trouble & Strife*, **2**, 10–17

Hobson D (1978) Housewives: isolation as oppression. In Women's Studies Group, Centre for Contemporary Cultural Studies, Birmingham (eds) *Women take Issue*. London; Hutchinson

Kinsey A S, Pomeroy W B, Martin C E & Gebhard P H (1948) *Sexual Behaviour in the Human Male*. Philadelphia: W B Saunders

Kinsey A S, Pomeroy W B, Martin C E & Gebhard P H (1953) *Sexual Behaviour in the Human Female*. Philadelphia: W B Saunders

Larrain J (1979) *The Concept of Ideology*. London: Hutchinson

Lennane K J & Lennane R J (1982) Alleged psychogenic disorders in women. A possible manifestation of sexual prejudice. In Whitelegg E et al. (eds) *The Changing Experience of Women*. Oxford: Martin Robertson/Open University

Masters W H & Johnson V E (1966) *Human Sexual Response*. Boston: Little Brown & Co

Melody G F (1962) Depressive reactions following hysterectomy. *American Journal of Obstetrics & Gynecology*, **83** (3), 410–413

Menzer D, Morris T, Gates P, Sabbath J, Robey H, Plant T & Sturgis S H (1957) Patterns of emotional recovery from hysterectomy. *Psychosomatic Medicine*, **19**, 379

Mitchell J & Oakley A (eds) (1976) *The Rights and Wrongs of Women*. Harmondsworth: Penguin Books

Nuttall P (1983) Male takeover or female giveaway? *Nursing Times*, **79** (2), 10–11

Oakley A (1981) *Subject Women*. Glasgow: Fontana

Patterson R M & Craig J B (1963) Psychological effects of hysterectomy. *American Journal of Obstetrics and Gynecology*, **85** (1), 104–111

Polivy J (1975) Psychological reactions to hysterectomy: a critical review. *American Journal of Obstetrics & Gynecology*, **111** (3), 417–426

Pollock L & West E (1984) On being a woman and a psychiatric nurse. *Senior Nurse*, **1** (17), 10–13

Rugen H *Women on the borderline of pathology: Dominant Conceptions of Female Sexuality in Health and Illness 1900–1920*. Unpublished paper, Science Studies Unit, University of Edinburgh

Raphael B (1972) The crisis of hysterectomy. *Australia & New Zealand Journal of Psychiatry*, **6**, 106–115

Richards D H (1973) Depression after hysterectomy. *The Lancet*, **2**, 430–432

Richardson A C & Lyon J B (1981) The prevention of post-operative infection in abdominal hysterectomy. *Clinical Obstetrics & Gynecology*, **24** (4), 1259

Scully D (1980) *Men who Control Women's Health. The Miseducation of Obstetrician-Gynecologists*. Boston: Houghton Mifflin

Scully D & Bart P (1973) A funny thing happened on the way to the orifice: women in gynecology textbooks. In Huber J (ed) *Changing Women in a Changing Society*. Chicago: University of Chicago Press

Steiner M & Aleksandrowicz D R (1970) Psychiatric sequelae to gynaecological operations. *Israel Annals of Psychiatry*, **8** (2), 186–192

Versluysen M C (1980) Old wives' tales? Women healers in English history. In Davies C (ed) *Rewriting Nursing History*. London: Croom Helm

Webb C & Wilson-Barnett J (1983) Coping with hysterectomy. *Journal of Advanced Nursing*, **8**, 311–319

Chapter 4

SOME OF THE ISSUES OF CHILDBIRTH

Ann M Thomson

Most of the care in childbirth in the United Kingdom is provided within the hospital part of the National Health Service, and very little in the community. It has been said that the 'system has taken over childbirth': if it has, it is incumbent upon the system to provide the best quality of care because the results of poor care have far-reaching effects.

Mortality rates in childbirth

Twentieth-century concern for reproduction has mostly centred on the topics of maternal* and perinatal† mortality. As a result of improvement in the physical health of women in general and changes which followed the systematic enquiry into the causes of maternal deaths engendered by the Confidential Enquiries into Maternal Mortality (DHSS 1982), childbirth in the United Kingdom is very safe for women in the 1980s. However, perinatal mortality is still giving some cause for concern. Although it is stated in the latest government report on Perinatal and Neonatal Mortality (DHSS 1984) that 'The perinatal mortality rate has fallen, is falling and can be expected to fall further' there are two riders: firstly, although the rate has fallen it still lags behind that of other countries, particularly those of Scandinavia; and secondly, 'Regional rates vary widely and social class differences remain and if anything may be increasing'.

---

* Maternity mortality = death of a woman from causes attributed to pregnancy and/or childbirth
† Perinatal mortality = death of a baby after the 28th week of gestation up to and including the first week of life.

There are some points which need consideration. The perinatal mortality rate has fallen from 15.5 deaths per 1,000 births in 1978 to 11.3 in 1982. One of the four suggested causes is a reduction in the number of notified births of babies with neural tube defects (DHSS 1984). The fact that fewer babies are being born with neural tube defects does not mean that fewer babies are also being conceived with these defects. With current facilities for assessing antenatal alpha-feto protein levels, ultrasound scanning and amniocentesis, a large number of babies who would have come within the perinatal mortality statistics are now featuring in the abortion statistics. Although it seems to be less distressing for the health professionals if these babies are not born, the distress caused to the parents is no less than if a perinatal death had occurred (Borg & Lasker 1982).

Secondly, is it right to compare British mortality rates with those of Scandinavia? Baird (1980) compared the perinatal mortality rates of Sweden with those of Scotland from the late 19th century to the present time and he demonstrated that although the rates were comparable at the beginning of this century the Scottish rates begun to lag behind those of Sweden in the depression of 1926–1937 (Sweden had no depression). On further examination of the statistics, and in particular those of neural tube defects, Baird demonstrated that the reproductive capability of those women conceived and born during the depression was adversley affected and resulted in the increased baby death rate from anencephaly which occurred in the late 1940s and 1950s. He thus suggests that environmental and socio-economic factors have a part to play in perinatal mortality. This point ties in with the second concern of the Short Report (DHSS 1984) that regional variations and differences between socio-economic groups still exist. Can the current economic recession be having an effect on perinatal mortality?

Causes of perinatal mortality

What are the causes of perinatal mortality? McIlwaine *et al.* (1979) carried out a retrospective analysis of the case records of all perinatal deaths occuring in Scotland in 1977. The three major causes of death were
- low birth weight (of normally-formed babies)
- fetal deformities
- antepartum haemorrhage.

Contributions to these causes are multifactorial but it is accepted that one of these causes of low birth weight is smoking after the twentieth week of gestation. It has been suggested that one of the possible causes of fetal deformity is dietary deficiency, in particular of amino acids, certain vitamins and trace elements, at the time of conception, and that one of the causes of antepartum haemorrhage is poor nutrition. If this is so, until women stop smoking in pregnancy and follow a nutritious diet the maternity services will be fighting an uphill battle in attempting to reduce the perinatal mortality rate.

There is evidence to suggest that a large proportion of women do stop smoking in early pregnancy, but what do we do to help the rest who find it difficult to abandon or even reduce the habit? It could be argued that we do very little. Black (1982) has suggested that we should:

(a) *ask each woman to try to cut down the number of cigarettes she smokes each day.* If she cannot do this we should

(b) *ask her to take five puffs per cigarette instead of 10* and, as the greatest concentration of nicotine and tar is in the last third of the cigarette,

(c) *ask her to leave a long stub.* We should suggest that she

(d) *always has an ashtray by her* and *should consciously put the cigarette down between puffs* as she is more likely to smoke if holding the cigarette. We should also

(e) *ask the woman to wait 10 minutes each time she feels the need to smoke* – eventually she will smoke fewer cigarettes each day. But what about the woman whose only prop is smoking? If we take away that prop what do we put in its stead?

As already stated, the quality of nutrition is thought to have some relationship with perinatal mortality. Durward (1984) asked the Home Economics Department at Salford College of Technology to prepare a week's menus for a pregnant woman based on dietary information given to women at maternity hospitals. The menus were then costed in nine areas in Great Britain. The average cost was £13.87, ranging from £13.46 in Cambridge to £14.30 in Oxfordshire. Durward (1984) points out that this takes 9% of average earnings, as in February 1984, but that for those on lower incomes the percentage is greater. The families who are in greatest difficulty are those receiving Supplementary Benefit where the cost of this diet can represent 32% of the basic allowance (excluding housing costs). The person who is in gravest difficulty is the single woman: the cost of her adequate diet takes 49% of her allowance and leaves her 'only £13.70 for fuel, clothing, transport and all other goods and service' (Durward, 1984).

Perinatal mortality is greatest in the lower socio-economic groups (Townsend & Davidson 1982; Cole et al. 1983; MacFarlane & Mugford 1984; DHSS 1984). It is the lower socioeconomic groups who have the lower incomes, who are more likely to be eligible for Family Income Supplement or, if not working, Supplementary Benefit. If the allowances are insufficient to enable a woman to buy food to give herself an adequate diet when pregnant what does this nation think of its future children? What have the maternity services to build on?

Where care is provided

Government reports since the 1920s have recommended that an increasing percentage of confinements should take place in hospital. It was the Peel Report (DHSS 1970) which recommended that ' . . . sufficient facilities should be provided to allow for 100% hospital delivery. The greater safety of hospital confinement for mother and child justifies this objective'. Tew (1978) has challenged this latter statement saying that there just are not the data to support it. Campbell et al. (1984) would appear to support this view. In a retrospective analysis of 'booked' home confinements occuring in 1979 they found a perinatal mortality rate (PNMR) of 4.1 per 1000 births, less than a third of the national rate. Campbell et al. also demonstrated that the PNMR for those delivering at home but not 'booked' for home confinement was 67.5 per 1000 births.

This is a vast difference. Previous analyses of the rates of death following home confinement have considered all the deaths together. Those women 'booked' to have a home confinement would, on the whole, have been those at least risk of mortality. Those with an unplanned home confinement were those women with a concealed pregnancy, or where everything happened too quickly for transfer to hospital. These two groups of women are different in their reproductive capability and, as Campbell et al. point out, when considering mortality rates for home confinement it is important to know where the confinements were planned to occur.

Even before publication of the Peel Report the percentage, in

1968, of births in hospital was 80.7. With confinement occuring in hospital, the meaning of childbirth has altered: it is now seen as a pathological event and not as a physiological one occuring naturally as part of the life cycle.

The maternity services provide antenatal care (which includes screening and education), care during labour and for delivery, and postnatal care.

Antenatal care

Oakley (1984) has pointed out that although J W Ballantyne is generally considered to be the father of antenatal care there was an international antenatal care movement which moved differently in different places. Oakley (1984) reports that Ballantyne stated in 1902 that 'Prevention in order to be truly preventive must be antenatal'. The Short Report (DHSS 1984) is of that view eighty years later when it says 'Antenatal care is a perfect example of preventive medicine'. The aim of antenatal care is to: prevent problems which might be avoided by prophylactic measures, to predict problems which may occur, and to treat conditions which may be harmful to mother and/or baby.

'Antenatal care in Britain has three major components-

1. Routine care administered to asymptomatic women according to an agreed pattern.
2. Education, information and reassurance for the pregnant woman,
3. Outpatient or inpatient care for specific problems such as haemorrhage, pain or sickness'. (Hall 1984)

For the woman to obtain this care she has to attend her general practitioner who will then refer her to a maternity unit: she cannot refer herself of her own volition. At the first so called 'booking clinic' she will be put on what can seem to be a conveyor belt which slowly moves her round a usually crowded, cramped clinic, through the hands of a large number of uniformed people, who do not introduce themselves or explain their status and their role. The woman is asked a bewildering number of questions which seem to have little relevance to the birth of her baby and some of which are repeated by many of the uniformed people. She will receive an equally bewildering amount of information both verbally and in leaflet form. The woman is given a physical examination, and in some hospitals this is split into two parts with one person examining the 'top' and another the 'bottom'. At the end of an average of two-and-a-half hours the woman is out on the street wondering just what has happened to her.

Subsequent visits for antenatal care are made monthly until the 28th week of gestation, fortnightly until the 36th week and weekly thereafter until delivery – that is, provided no abnormality occurs. However, this has meant that a large number of women attend a clinic and have to wait on average for two hours to be seen by a doctor (and not the same doctor each time) for two minutes. The women have rightly expressed their dissatisfaction (Garcia 1982) and have asked What is this care? As MacIntyre (1984) points out, the sad thing about the complaints that are made is that they are the same in the 1980s as they were in the 1940s. All working women now have the right to reasonable paid time off work for antenatal care (Employment Act 1980). But is the hospital aware of the antagonism of an employer towards antenatal care caused to by a three-hour absence from production by an employee?

When childbirth was taken into the hospital the 'good bits' about home confinement were not taken in as well. Doctors (in this case, obstetricians) are in charge in hospital so everything is done for their convenience. Because doctors are regarded as busy people, antenatal clinic staff will have women lined up (without knickers and tights) ready to be examined so that the greatest number of pregnant tums can be looked at in the shortest amount of time. This practice has led to complaints that antenatal care is de-humanising and raises anxiety levels because questions are not answered.

There is a failure in hospital antenatal clinics to understand the basics of communication. Women are required to lie flat on their backs, so that not only are they in a vulnerable position but the doctor is in a superior one. Desks to hold the notes are positioned so that the only way the woman can look at the person at the desk is to screw her neck round at an angle of 90° and look up at the same time – not the most comfortable position when you are 38-weeks pregnant. Graham & Oakley (1977) found that obstetricians did not like to discover women sitting up on the couch when they came into the cubicle but that it was these women who obtained most information. However, MacIntyre (1984) suggests that the problems of communication in antenatal clinics are due to problems of 'doctor-patient communication in general rather than in antenatal care alone'.

During recent years it has been recognised that it is unnecessary for all women to attend hospital for all their antenatal check-ups. A system of 'shared-care' has been introduced whereby the GP undertakes some or all of the care. The schemes vary from area to area – in some the woman only returns to the hospital for delivery, in others the GP sees her until the 32nd week and then hands her over to the hospital. The idea behind 'shared care' is that the greater proportion of women are normal and can therefore be looked after by the GP, and it is better if the woman receives continuity of care from a health professional she knows well. The theory of this is good but the practice does not always live up to the ideal. Gutteridge (1981) found that women could see just as many doctors in the 'shared care scheme' as they would have done if they had received care at the hospital and that the quality of care provided was sadly lacking in some cases.

Schemes have been set-up whereby antenatal care is taken to women in the community. The three most famous schemes are those in Lambeth (Zander *et al.* 1978; Taylor 1984), the East End of Glasgow (Reid *et al.* 1983) and the Sighthill project in Edinburgh (McKee 1984). None of the schemes has been shown to have a detrimental effect on the outcome of pregnancy. Some have shown a reduction in the defaulters rate (McKee 1984; Taylor 1984) and one (McKee 1984) has shown a reduction in the perinatal mortality rate of the women attending the clinic over that of women living in the area but attending the hospital for antenatal care. This last clinic does not allow women to default: if it is thought that attendance at the clinic will be too difficult for them their antenatal care is then provided at home.

As a spin off from these new community clinics, women now carry their own medical records (these are more detailed than the 'co-op card'), so that the notes are readily available in the antenatal clinic and when the women are admitted to hospital in labour. Critics of this system say that it is unprofessional for women to hold their confidential notes because they will read them and lose them. Experience has shown that notes are available more often than when held in medical records departments, and that the women do read their notes – some even contribute to them, and enjoy the demystification of their pregnancy (Murray & Topley 1974; Taylor 1984).

Women are not the only group of people who are dissatisfied with antenatal care. Obstetricians have been questioning the cost effectiveness of antenatal care as it is currently provided. Chng *et al*. (1980) and Hall *et al*. (1980) undertook a retrospective analysis of the notes of the women who delivered in Aberdeen in 1975. They found that obstetricians were not as vigilant as midwives in noting potential medical problems, that women with potential problems were 'booked' inappropriately for confinement in peripheral units, and that intra-uterine growth retardation was only detected in 44% of cases and overdiagnosed by a factor of 2.5. Hall *et al*, (1980) suggest that it is not necessary to see women as often as is currently the practice and that it is not necessary to carry out all the rituals at every visit.

Labour and delivery

When it was the case that women had their babies at home they were in their own surroundings, and the health professionals who came to assist them were guests and could only enter by invitation. In hospital, the doctors and midwives are in charge – it is their domain, which means that women are unable to remain in control of their own labour and delivery. On admission to a delivery unit, a woman is stripped of her identity by the removal of her clothes, she is given an institutional nightdress, and she has to put a small number of belongings into a plastic bag – the rest have to be taken home in her suitcase. In case she forgets who she is she is given a plastic bracelet with her name on it.

Even though research has shown that routine vulval shaving (Romney 1980) and the giving of enemas in labour have no value (Romney & Gordon 1981; Drayton & Rees 1983) there are still some maternity units which routinely subject women to these degrading procedures. Once it has been ascertained that the woman is established in labour she is moved into a labour room and connected up to a fetal monitor which effectively ties her to the bed.

When women delivered their babies at home they remained

up and mobile for the greater proportion of the labour and carried on with household chores until they felt the need to retire to bed. Their surroundings were familiar, there was plenty of distraction from the pain of contractions, and they were not separated from the family. The amount of analgesia they used was small in comparison to that used in hospital and the midwife looking after them was the one who carried out the antenatal care.

In the 1980s the labour ward midwives are strangers to the labouring women. There is very little distraction for women in the labour ward, beds are notoriously hard and uncomfortable, and medical equipment in the room does not always engender a feeling of tranquility. There have been attempts to humanise labour wards. Walls have been painted in non-institutionalised colours, wallpaper has even been hung, curtains have been put up, bean bags, soft cushions and floor mats have been provided, and rocking chairs have added a touch of home: however, all these refurbishments are of no use if the attitudes of the attendants are inappropriate.

Some authorities have set up 'birthing rooms', decorated and furnished similarly to a bedroom at home. These rooms are available for use by those women the obstetric staff have predicted will have a normal labour and delivery. Whatever equipment might be needed is hidden behind curtains or in cupboards. This is a nice idea, but what happens to those women not allowed to use a birthing room? How do they feel when they are told that their delivery is potentially too dangerous to use these homely facilities. Surely women who have medical and/or obstetric abnormalities should not be subjected to the added stress of unattractive surroundings, surgical equipment visible in glass cupboards, and an uncomfortable bed to which they are 'tied'. But are birthing rooms safer than home, because if hospital is safer, as claimed by the Peel Report (DHSS 1970), then it is so because of the availability of facilities. If the full facilities are not readily available some women might then be safer having a home confinement.

Research undertaken with animals has demonstrated that if they are disturbed in labour the labour stops until the disturbance has ceased. Although it is unwise to extrapolate directly from animals to humans it seems strange that labour ward staff have not recognised that the constant entering of labour ward rooms by anyone and everyone from the cleaner to the consultant, the ward clerk to the student midwife might have a disruptive effect on the labouring woman. It is not just physical intrusion into the room which disturbs but also the surreptitious lifting of the curtain over the window in the door, or the slight opening of the venetian blinds, both varieties of invasion of privacy.

Because of the concern with perinatal mortality, obstetricians have placed great emphasis on supervision and monitoring of the mother and fetus during labour. The supervision has taken the form of an invasion, by obstetricians, of the labour ward. In some units the invasion has become a 'round' of each labouring woman morning and evening by the consultant and his entourage: this can mean as many as 15 people entering a labour room at one time. Patients in general wards have complained about this type of treatment – they feel like animals in the zoo, especially when doctors talk over the top of them, so how much worse must it be for women experiencing the intermittent pain of contractions? Monitoring the mother and fetus during labour has, in some units, taken the form of routine continuous monitoring, that is, all women have a transducer recording uterine activity and an electrode on the fetal scalp recording the heartbeat. Women have complained because being attached to a machine reduces their mobility and they are concerned about the potential for damage to their baby by the scalp electrode. MacDonald *et al.* (1985) have demonstrated an increased instrumental delivery rate in a group of women monitored continuously in labour when compared with a group monitored intermittently. Is routine continuous montoring necessary? The World Health Organisation thinks not as it states:

> 'There is no evidence that routine intrapartum electronic fetal monitoring has a positive effect on the outcome of pregnancy.' (WHO 1985)

In the 1970s, a great debate raged in the midwifery and obstetric world as a result of the writing and sayings of Frederick Leboyer (1975). Once the initial storm had calmed down it was realised that perhaps he had a point – we were being violent to newborn babies, we were handling them unkindly with our hands, with light and with noise. More recently Michel Odent (1984) has created another storm. In his unit in Pithiviers (France), women labour in rooms decorated in warm, earthy colours, there is no clock, there is a minimum of constraining furniture, a warm bath is available if necessary, the woman is disturbed as little as possible and analgesia is not given. The critics of Odent state that there is very little science to back up his sayings and that the statistics from his unit are very difficult to understand because socio-economic details are not available. Odent's critics may be right but there is certainly a lot of art in what he practices. Perhaps what we need is a marriage of the art and the science. There are some women, however, who do not like Odent's practice of no analgesia – they want to know that it is available should they want it – it's a question of choice.

In 1982, a conference entitled Active Birth was held at the Wembley conference centre in London – over 2,000 people attended. The conference participants were mothers, fathers, babies, pregnant women, midwives, antenatal teachers, obstetricians, GPs, paediatricians, and epidemiologists. The participants were there to learn and share their experiences of Active Birth. The factors which contribute to Active Birth are preparation for childbirth, both physical and psychological, surroundings where the woman can be in control, where she is not tied to a bed and where she can adapt her position to what her body wants her to do.

The physiological position for labour is upright because the fetal presenting part is then brought into close contact with the cervix: this provides reflex stimulation to the contractions and the pelvis can 'give' as the fetus descends. If the woman is lying on her back the presenting part of the fetus is not in close contact with the cervix and the sacrum cannot move back because the woman is lying on it. The pain of the contractions is also greater when the woman is lying down.

The upright position for labour and delivery is not a new fad of the 1980s. It is well documented that women were required to take to their beds for labour in the seventeenth century when doctors (male, of course) became interested in childbirth: they could not care for a woman on a birthing stool. Russell (1982) and Hillan (1983) have demonstrated that women in so called 'primitive societies' used a variety of methods and pieces of equipment to maintain a vertical posture in labour, and Russell (1969) has shown that a squatting position for delivery can increase the available pelvic outlet by as much as 20–30%. Could it be that the practice of discouraging mobility in labour and therefore not taking advantage of the effects of gravity can have contributed to the rise in the Caesarean section rate as described by Boyd & Francome (1983).

The perineum has received much attention in the medical press in the past two decades. Obstetricians, who are also gynaecologists, were concerned because of the apparently large number of women referred to them with vaginal prolapse and stress incontinence. They, the obstetricians, surmised that this was due to excessive stretching during childbirth and that one way to prevent this was to undertake routine elective episiotomy. Women have questioned the need for routine episiotomy because of the side effects, namely perineal pain and dyspareunia. The protagonists of episiotomy claim that because it is a clean cut it heals more efficiently, while the antagonists claim that an episiotomy is more painful postnatally than a tear. Sleep et al. (1984) conducted a randomised controlled trial to assess the benefits and hazards of episiotomy. The subjects (1000) were allocated either to a group where an episiotomy was to be restricted as far as possible to fetal indications only, or to a group where spontaneous perineal trauma was to be prevented. Three months after delivery there was no difference in the incidence of perineal pain, resumption of sexual intercourse, dyspareunia and incontinence between the two groups; this was in spite of the fact that there was a 10.2% incidence of episiotomy in the group where it was to be restricted and 51.4% in the group where spontaneous trauma was to be prevented. Sleep et al. state that restricting the operation increases the number of women who deliver without trauma and that 'in the absence of positive proof that this invasive procedure is of benefit to the mother it may be suggested that the rationale for practice is in need of drastic reappraisal'. The third stage of labour (the time when the placenta is delivered) has also been subject to interventions. Inch (1985) has, by undertaking an extensive literature review, demonstrated that the effects of one intervention have led to the need for another, and then another. She questions the need for any intervention in the third stage of labour unless it is vital for the mother's health.

Postnatal care

The postnatal period is the time when the mother recovers physically and emotionally from the pain and work of labour. It is the time when both parents should be getting to know their new baby and learning to care for her. To be able to do this requires rest, a good diet, privacy and continuity of care from health professionals: this is virtually impossible to obtain in hospital, as ably described by McHardy (1984). Provided they have adequate housekeeping facilities it would be far better if the greater proportion of delivered women were transferred home within 24 hours of delivery. At home the woman (and her baby) will control when she eats and sleeps, she will be able to control the temperature of her environment, she will be able to have visitors when convenient to her and her diet will suit her tastes. If the woman is at home the community midwife will provide all the midwifery care, if she is in hospital only a small proportion will be provided by a midwife – the rest will be provided by auxiliary nurses, nursery nurses, student nurses and enrolled nurses.

Breast feeding is a subject which appears to engender either love or hate. Currently in Britain, there are two generations of women who have had no experience of breast feeding: there are two generations of midwives who have not assisted women to breast feed. Fisher (1985) has demonstrated that at the beginning of this century paediatricians were thought to be expert in the new techniques of feeding babies other than by the breast. These experts then applied the principles of bottle feeding to the practice of breast feeding. The two do not mix because the physiology of lactation is that supply is controlled by demand and if demand is restricted, eg. by controlling the frequency of feeds, or attempting to control their length or by giving complementary cows milk feeds, then the supply will be inadequate. The frequency of feeds may need to be hourly or six-hourly depending on the baby's thirst and or hunger. It seems strange that adults eat sweets or biscuits and drink tea or coffee between meals but get upset if a baby tries to do that.

The midwife

So far there has been very little mention of the midwife. A

midwife in the UK is a woman (or man) trained to provide care for normal childbirth on her own responsibility. She is trained to recognise the abnormal and call in medical aid: where medical aid is not available she will provide the necessary care. With the move of childbirth into the hospital the role of the midwife has been diminished. Midwives have been relegated to the role of chaperones for obstetricians in antenatal clinics and to maternity nurses in labour wards. They were usually left in charge of postnatal wards but recent policy on staff grades and levels has meant that too much of the postnatal care has been left to people other than midwives. This has led to lack of job satisfaction and is said to be the cause of the shortage of midwives that Robinson (1980) found.

However, there are signs that the midwife is at last waking up to her position, her voice is at last being heard. She is increasingly demanding and providing antenatal care and increasingly is taking responsibility for the care she provides in labour. One midwife is currently undertaking a research project where a team of midwives provide total care for childbirth for a group of women (Flint 1985). This means that not only are the women provided with continuity of care but the midwife sees childbirth in its total perspective.

The midwife has to learn to say who she is wherever she is working – too many people only recognise her if she is cycling to homes in the country. Thomson (1978) found that women receiving antenatal care in hospital denied all knowledge of speaking to a midwife and yet they had just been talking to her, they saw her as 'the nurse'. Leinster (1983) found this in the Newcastle Primary Health Care Project and states that 'midwives no longer have a clear identity to the public'.

Newson (1982) cautions us to take care over the kind of identity we present to the public when she states 'It must be slightly perplexing for a woman to be told the importance of good diet and abstinence from nicotine when her adviser is overweight, unfit and perhaps smells of cigarette smoke'. She is ably supported by Hazel and Helen:

'Hazel – Well, I mean, now, I'm overweight and when you look at T. she is very untidy, I mean, I am not being personal, but when you look at somebody you get that image. And to me, when she used to say 'Take a lot of notice of your post natal exercises' and I used to look at her and think: 'Well, you haven't, have you?' (laughs). I mean, she is as wide as she is tall.

Helen — No, when she was on about diet which is what she used to talk about most of the time, it was difficult to take her seriously.' (Leinster 1983, p 34)

Childbirth care in the community

With the removal of childbirth into hospital, responsibility for childbirth has been taken away from the community. In the introduction to *Health for a Change* Dowling (1983) states that one of the main aims of the NHS has not been achieved, that is that '*all* people should have equality of access to health care. The parents and young children who are most at risk from ill-health and premature death are still those for whom our preventive health services are least available and least used'. Dowling (1983) continues that 'The main place for the NHS's preventive health services must be in the community . . . ' Unfortunately not all authorities agree with this concept, eg. although reporting on the problem of heroin addiction a recent newspaper report quoted a health administrator as saying 'They (the local council) took the line that anyone who's ill should be treated in hospital, not in a shopping precinct'. Now, childbearing women are not ill, they are having a baby, but why can they not have facilities in the shopping precinct? Leinster (1984) asked women about the health care services that they wanted. By quoting the women verbatim she (Leinster) has given a richness to the report which is often lacking in other research reports: to try to summarise this removes the richness, but women want to be given the choice to decide where they will have their care and where they will deliver their babies, they want privacy when this care is being given, they do not want to be kept waiting, and they want facilities for their older children while the care is being given.

The Child Poverty Action Group undertook a project which was designed to attempt to map out new developments in the way preventive care in pregnancy and early childhood is provided (Dowling 1983). There are places where walk-in pregnancy care facilities exist in the centre of town. Employers are cooperating in providing health education and counselling for pregnant and non-pregnant employees. Some areas have set up 'out-of-hours' health promotion services staffed by midwives and health visitors.

Some members of the health professions are of the opinion that childbirth cannot occur 'safely' without a massive input from the health service agencies, with the service centred on the hospital. But if, the main problems are social in origin (Townsend & Davidson 1982; Cole *et al*. 1983; MacFarlane & Mugford 1984; DHSS 1984), what can the hospital hope to do? Although major advances have been made in the antenatal detection of congenital abnormalities, such as neural tube defects, further efforts need to be concentrated on the prevention of these defects. Hall *et al*. (1980) have questioned the value of the large number of visits women are required to make to the antenatal clinic and there is certainly a need for a re-appraisal of the effects and benefits of antenatal care as it is currently provided. In the light of the work of Campbell *et al*. (1984), the 100% hospital confinement policy in this country should be re-examined. With current concerns about the cost of the National Health Service both the emotional and financial costs of current provision of postnatal care would benefit from examination: surely it would be much better to assess each woman individually on her need to remain in hospital? Although there will always be a need for specialised care in childbirth for some women, the number requiring this will be relatively small; rationalisation of facilities is needed so that the specialists providing care can concentrate their efforts with such women and not try to spread themselves over all childbearing women. This would mean returning the care of normal childbearing women to midwives – both community and hospital. Finally, it would appear that the greatest reduction in mortality statistics could be achieved if childbearing women were able to provide themselves with an adequate diet. Society has to decide if it is willing to provide the means to buy an adequate diet to those least able to feed themselves, namely those in the lower socio-economic groups.

References

Baird D (1980) Environment and reproduction. *British Journal of Obstetrics and Gynaecology*, **87**(12), 1057–1567

Ballantyne J W (1902) *Manual of Antenatal Pathology and Hygiene. Vol 1.* Edinburgh: William Green & Sons

Black P M (1982) *The effects of low tar cigarettes on birthweight.* Proceedings of the Research and the Midwife Conference

Borg S & Lasker J (1982) *When Pregnancy Fails. Coping with Miscarriage, Stillbirth and Infant Death.* London: Routledge & Kegan Paul

Boyd C & Francome C (1983) *One Birth in Nine, Caesarean Sections Trends since 1978.* London: Maternity Alliance

Campbell R, MacDonald, Davies I, McFarlane A & Beral V (1984) Home Births in England and Wales, 1979. Perinatal Mortality according to intended place of delivery. *British Medical Journal*, **289** (6447), 721–724

Chng P K, Hall M & MacGillivray I (1980) An Audit of Antenatal Care: The value of the first antenatal visit. *British Medical Journal*, **281** (6249) 1184–1186

Cole T J, Donnet M L & Stanfield S P (1983) Unemployment, birthweight growth in the first year. *Archives of Disease in Childhood*, **58**, 717–721

DHSS (1970) *Domiciliary Midwifery and Maternity Bed Needs. (The Peel Report).* London: HMSO

DHSS (1982) *Report on Confidential Enquiries into Maternal Deaths in England and Wales, 1976–1978.* London HMSO

DHSS (1984) *Perinatal and Neonatal Mortality – Follow up (Short Report).* London: HMSO

Dowling S (1983) *Health for a Change. The Provision of Preventive Health Care in Pregnancy and Early Childhood.* London: Child Poverty Action Group

Drayton S, Rees C (1983) They know what they're doing. The midwife and enemas. *Proceedings of 1983 Research and the Midwife Conference*

Durward L (1984) *Poverty in Pregnancy, the Cost of an Adequate Diet for Expectant Mothers.* London: Maternity Alliance

Fisher C (1985) How did we go wrong with breast feeding? Midwifery, **1** (1). 48–51

Flint C (1985) Labour of love. *Nursing Times*, Jan 30, 16–18

Garcia J (1982) Women's views of antenatal care. In Enkin M & Chalmers I (eds) *Effectiveness and Satisfaction in Antenatal Care.* London: Spastics International Medical Publications

Graham H & Oakley A (1977) *Competing Ideologies of Reproduction: Medical and Maternal Perspectives on Pregnancy and Childbirth.* Paper presented at the Second Seminar on Human Relations, in Obstetric Practice, Warwick University, July

Gutteridge S (1981) General practitioner care. Paper presented at *Human Relations and Obstetric Problems Conference, Glasgow* – Reproduced in Reid M E, Gutteridge S & McIlwaine G M (1982). *A Comparison of the Delivery of Antenatal Care between a Hospital and a Peripheral Clinic.* Social Paediatric and Obstetric Research Unit, University of Glasgow

Hall M (1984) Are our accepted practices based on valid assumptions. In

Zander L & Chamberlain G (eds) *Pregnancy Care for the 1980s*. London; Royal Society of Medicine, Macmillan Press

Hall M, Chng P K & MacGillivray, I. (1980) Is routine antenatal care worthwhile? *Lancet*, **2** (8185), 78–80

HMSO (1980) *Employment Act*. London: HMSO

Hillan E (1983) *The Birthing Chair Trial*. Proceedings of Research and the Midwife Conference

Inch S (1985) Management of the third stage of labour – a cascade of intervention? *Midwifery*, **1** (2)

Leboyer F (1975) *Birth Without Violence*. London: Wildwood House

Leinster C (1983) *What we need is . . . Women; Health and the Health Service in Newcastle-upon-Tyne*. Newcastle-upon-Tyne Inner City Forum

MacDonald D, Grant A, Sheridan-Pereira M, Boylan P & Chalmers I (1985) The Dublin randomized controlled trial of intrapartum fetal heart rate monitoring. *American Journal of Obstetrics and Gynacology*, **152**, 524–537

MacFarlane A & Mugford M (1984) *Birth Counts*. London: HMSO

McHardy A (1984) The joys of a special delivery. *Guardian*, Sept 24, 11

McIlwaine G, Howat R C L, Dunn F & MacNaughton MC (1979) *Scotland 1977 Perinatal Mortality Survey*. University of Glasgow: Department of Obstetrics and Gynacology

MacIntyre S (1984) Consumer reaction to present-day antenatal services. In Zander L & Chamberlain G (eds) *Pregnancy Care for the 1980s*. London: Royal Society of Medicine Macmillan Press

McKee I H (1984) Community antenatal care: the Sighthill Community Antenatal Scheme. In Zander L & Chamberlain G (eds) *Pregnancy Care for the 1980s*. London: Royal Society of Medicine Macmillan Press

Murray FA & Topley L (1974) Patients as record holders. *Health and Social Services Journal*, **84** (4397), 1675

Newson K (1982) The future of midwifery. *Midwife, Health Visitor and Community Nurse*, **18**, 528–532

Oakley A (1984) *The Captured Womb*. Oxford: Basil Blackwell

Odent M (1984) *Entering the World. The De-medicalisation of Childbirth*. London: Marion Boyers

Reid M Gutteridge S & McIlwaine G M (1982) *A Comparison of the Delivery of Antenatal Care between a Hospital and a Peripheral Clinic*. University of Glasgow: Social Paediatric and Obstetric Research Unit.

Robinson S (1980) *Midwifery Manpower, NERU Occasional Paper No. 4*. London University: Nursing Education Research Unit

Romney M (1980) *Pre-delivery Shaving: An Unjustified Assault*. Proceedings of 1979 and 1980 Research and the Midwife Conference

Romney M Gordon (1981) Is your enema really necessary? *British Medical Journal*, **282** (18/4), 1269

Russell J G B (1969) Moulding of the pelvic outlet. *Journal of Obstetrics and Gynaecology of the British Commonwealth*, **76**, 817–829

Russell J C B (1982) The Rationale of Primitive Delivery Positions. *British Journal of Obstetrics and Gynaecology, London*, **89**, 712–715

Sleep J, Grant A, Garcia J, Elbourne D, Spencer J & Chalmers I (1984) West Berkshire Perineal Management Trial. *British Medical Journal*, **289**, 587–590

Taylor R W (1984) Community-based Specialist Obstetric Services. In Zander L & Chamberlain G (eds) *Pregnancy Care for the 1980s*. London: Royal Society of Medicine Macmillan Press

Tew M (1978) The Case Against Hospital Deliveries: The Statistical Evidence. In Kitzinger S & Davis J A (eds) *The Place of Birth*. Oxford University Press

Thomson A M (1978) *Why don't Woman Breast Feed?* Unpublished Report to Scottish Home and Health Department, Edinburgh

Townsend P & Davidson N (1982) *Inequalities in Health, The Black Report*, Harmondsworth: Penguin Books

WHO (1985) *Appropriate Technology for Birth. Report of the Joint EURO/ PAHO Working Group*. World Health Organisation

Zander L, Watson M, Taylor R & Morrell D G (1978) Integration of general practitioner and specialist antenatal care. *Journal of Royal College of General Practitioners*, **28**, 455

Chapter 5

WOMEN AND MENTAL HEALTH

Lorraine Smith

Since the late sixties, the women's movement has forced the examination of many entrenched ideas. It has struggled to establish equal rights for women regarding employment and pay. It has highlighted the difficulties that women experience isolated in their own homes. The conflicts created from the many roles women are expected to fulfil have also found expression through the women's movement, and perhaps, more importantly, the basic asymmetry of male-female relationships in Western society has been disclosed.

The field of mental helth is as representative as any other in failing to come to terms with the issues and stresses that confront women. A recommendation that psychiatrists include in their education and treatment planning, a knowledge and understanding of the goals, aspirations and writings of the women's movement has seldom been implemented in the U K (Editorial, *American Journal of Psychiatry 1981*).

Yet it is with concern that it must be pointed out that most psychiatrists are male, that most psychiatrists see female patients, that a much larger proportion of psychiatric and medical patients are female and, finally, that the most common problem women face is depression, approximately two-thirds of all depressed patients being female.

It is therefore worrying indeed that most women will be treated by men who may have little perception of the dilemma of a woman's everyday existence. Furthermore, psychiatrists are no less immune to the traditional beliefs and values of Western society concerning a woman's place. It can be anticipated that they will reflect these views in any interpretation of female behaviour.

Mental health professionals tend to concentrate on internal processes in developing theories about behaviour, largely ignoring external factors which realistically might contribute to a far greater understanding of a woman's state of mind. A woman is supposed to be happy, to feel fulfilled, to be content in her assigned roles of mother and wife: if, in fact, she is unhappy, discontented, despairing or experiences resentment and anger, it is she, the woman, who is at fault, not her situation. Therein lies a paradox. The woman who feels she is to blame for her unhappiness is at the same time unable to exert sufficient control over herself to alter her state of misery. The dilemma is complete, for not only is she to blame but she is also powerless to alter circumstances. It is of little wonder that women frequently describe themselves as 'trapped'.

A chapter such as this can only scratch the surface. In view of this, two major themes have been selected from which it is hoped that a greater understanding of women will be derived. The first theme is that of role conflict with its accompanying experience of stress. The other major theme is loss. Various coping mechanisms are described which might go some way to explaining how women currently manage dissonance in their lives. In concluding the chapter, some suggestions are put forward for changing and gaining control of one's life.

Stress and marriage

Stress

Stress can be seen as any influence either from within an individual or arising from pressures in the environment which interfere or prevent basic needs being met, or disrupt, or threaten to disrupt, that individual's homeostatic balance. Thus, we can see that stress occurs in many guises such as self-criticism, illness or too many demands on ourselves and our time and resources.

Broadly speaking, stress may be divided into three principal categories. The first is concernced with loss, or a threat of loss, to aspects of ourselves which we hold to be important or significant. These might include personal relationships, status, body function and body image. The second major category centres on actual or threatened injury to our bodies. Connected with injury are the notions of pain and mutilation: most of us fear pain and take care to prevent injury to our person. When we are injured we experience stress as we wait to learn how the injury will influence our lives. Frustration of the basic biological drives constitutes the last category. Here we are talking about the need for shelter, warmth, group-belonging, food, sex, and so on: inability to satisfy these drives leads to stress. Included within this last category is the need for appropriate channels to dispel aggressive impulses; sporting and recreational activities are two examples of channels which might be employed.

In writing about stress Rapoport (1965) distinguishes between a stressful event and a crisis situation. A crisis is seen to have growth-promoting potential in that it causes an individual to adapt and search for new behaviours. It may, in fact, raise a person's level of mental health. Stress, on the other hand, is a subjective experience from which one emerges to survive or to crack under pressure. In this sense, stress is a negative life event in that it reduces one's level of mental health.

Adaptation to stress is a learned response; that is, as we encounter stressful situations we learn to minimise the discomfort experienced. Various approaches are attempted until one is hit upon which seems to be the most effective in relieving pressure.

Gillis (1972) suggests a variety of approaches which may be utilised to promote adaptation. These are as follows:
1. Direct action to deal with a problem in order to prevent, diminish or resolve it.
2. Mental withdrawal from the problem. Gillis believes that if this pattern of behaviour is used extensively it can lead to isolation, passivity, or extreme submissiveness.
3. Flight or physical removal of self from the problem.
4. Compensation or the acceptance of an alternative satisfaction.
5. Illness whereby psychosomatic symptoms represent a failure to adapt.
6. Repression in which the problem is unconsciously submerged in the mind.

Based on the preceding comments, it can be stated unequivocally that women have the potential to experience considerable stress in their lives. It is this potential for stress which will now be examined.

It seems to be almost inevitable that we marry. Societal pressure such as family continuity, succession, inheritance and security propel us towards the objective of marriage. Equally, the need to find fulfilment, happiness and companionship plays a part. Marriage is often prompted by the desire for children, and religion supports and reinforces this rationale. Marriage is one of the social norms in our society; to be married is to increase our self-esteem primarily because we are the object of desire. As people wryly admit, it is rather like joining a club.

Yet, today in Western society there exists a choice: no-one is compelled to marry. Safe and effective contraception means that children can be planned. Women have access to education and therefore possess the potential to support themselves. But still we marry, and not just once. If marriage proves disastrous the first time, we continue to experiment in the hope of discovering the winning formula of 'and they lived together happily for ever and ever'.

If one examines the facts pertaining to marriage it is apparent that the impact of marriage is far greater on women than men. This statement might seem somewhat incredible but let's look at the facts. Married women seek more help for physical and mental problems than either married men or single women; women who are housebound with young children experience the highest rates of depression; approximately two-thirds of the women with three children under the age of five are depressed: and unmarried women have lower rates of mental illness as compared with unmarried men.

The evidence suggests strongly that the state of marriage creates greater stress for women than men. We can speculate that traditional beliefs, values, and role expectations contribute to conflict in the married woman, thus producing high stress levels which may ultimately lead to depression or other health-seeking behaviours.

We must then return to the question as to why women marry. It is unlikely that women in the premarital period either know or believe that marriage may be deterimental to their health. It would seem that women are so enmeshed in the romantic tales that are spun regarding marriage that they are unable to detach themselves sufficiently to listen to their mothers, grandmothers and aunts who are older and perhaps wiser in the ways of the world. At the same time, mothers pass on to daughters their acquired wisdoms regarding men in the hope that their female children will be wary and 'guard themselves closely'.

Yet we do not have to marry; and until women grasp this reality they will continue to experience conflict. The capacity to make a choice and say 'I choose to marry' rather than 'I want to marry', or 'it's expected that I will marry', means that one enters marriage fully cogniscant of its realities and prepared to accept and exert responsibility.

Marriage

There is a tendency for women to be defined by their relationships to others, and to men in particular. Initially, you are your father's daughter; you move on to become someone's wife and eventually you are your children's mother. Very seldom are women introduced purely on their own merit. The fact that women require relationships in order to define their status implies that they have a poorly-developed self-identity, yet we know that the view one has of oneself is essential to establishing a personal sense of worth and value. If one's value is derived through others rather than through oneself, one is always at the mercy of how others perceive you.

Within marriage women are expected to fulfil many roles – wife, mother, homemaker and lover. A wife may also act as a social secretary, nurse and chauffeur, and probably works outside the home at some point in her marital life. Each role demands its own specific skills, but by and large they are skills which are not commercially viable.

Nadelson & Notman (1981) suggest three reasons why married women experience more stress than men. Firstly, they believe that marriage itself causes women to modify their lives more than it does for men, with a consequent loss of autonomy. Whilst acknowledging that this is changing, it is pointed out that change does not guarantee a reduction in stress.

It is usually the case that a man's career dictates the family life-style. If his job requires relocation, the family moves. The man, once installed in a new position, changes gear and carries on: a woman, on the other hand, must re-establish her connections. Friends that had acted as safety nets are no longer accessible. Instead, a woman must begin to rebuild a network, often through children, and if the children are older and she is no longer required to pick them up after school or transport them to various activities, her isolation may continue for some time. During this period her husband works, consorting within an already established system.

The second reason put forward by Nadelson & Notman (1981) to account for high female stress levels centres on the housewife's role. They note that the role is ascribed, not achieved, and although women perform well within it, there is no opportunity for diversification. Women feel the need to succeed in the homemaking role but as no criteria for success exist it is difficult to measure success. Without such criteria women may believe that they are failing.

Married women are cautioned not to bombard their husbands with the details of their day as soon as he walks in: after all, a man has been hard at work all day. Yet, the woman who spends an entire day with young children has almost certainly worked as hard as her husband and she may have had no opportunity to engage in adult conversation, read a paper or drink a cup of hot coffee. However, traditional beliefs regarding the role of housewife devalue her input; and women in turn accede to this devaluation.

Society does not value the homemaker role. It is unpaid labour; husbands generally do not insure against the loss of their wives' input; women refer to themselves as 'just housewives'. It is a dilemma, and it seems to make no difference whether one enjoys homemaking or not. If this is the experience of a woman, how can she derive a postive view of herself?

The loss of status incurred when a woman gives up her career to marry or have children is cited as a third source of stress. Status is a major contributor to self-esteem. Giving up one's career is a dramatic shift in focus and usually involves a sense of loss. Oft times the loss experienced by a woman is denigrated because her salary, as 'befits' most female occupations, is seen as contributory to the family income, not the mainstay. In addition, many of the so-called female occupations are not seen as career paths but simply as a means of biding time until marriage.

Women do experience loss in sublimating their job prospects to the perceived needs of the family. But again, women devalue their loss. It is ironic that women find themselves in a Catch 22 situation wherein they experience loss but as they have devalued the feelings they are then unable to communicate their experience because society of which they are a part, denies they ought to feel such a thing.

It is the woman who is both wife and mother and who is also employed outside the home who highlights the clash between traditional beliefs and recent attitudinal changes regarding a woman's place in the scheme of things. A constant juggling act is performed in the interests of striking a balance between homemaking tasks and the demands of the job.

Most working wives and mothers earn insufficient amounts to enable them to employ others to relieve them of some of the pressures involved in running a home. In such instances one would expect spouses to negotiate the housework and the care of the children: however, this is often not the case. Furthermore, working mothers may experience guilt regarding the care of the family and as a result may over-compensate by attempting to perform all those tasks they would normally engage upon if at home on a continuing basis. In addition, it is likely that they persist in making all the domestic arrangements, take time off from their employment to nurse sick children and adjust their work patterns to meet the needs of the family. The extent to which husbands recognise the stress created therein and are prepared to adapt their domestic life style is questionable.

It seems that while women are prepared to work to maintain their identity and make a contribution to the family income, they are unable to slay the ghosts of traditional values. Men, on the other hand, seldom experience similar stresses.

Loss

For many women loss can be viewed as a recurrent theme in their lives. Symbolic representation of this idea is found in the monthly event of menstruation which is colloquially referred to as a 'loss'.

Perhaps the first sense of loss women experience occurs shortly after puberty. The young girl is confronted by her own womanhood and sexuality: she may quietly mourn for her childhood. In many cultures the male child, having reached the age of thirteen or thereabouts, participates in a ritual which acknowledges and celebrates his manhood. The passage from girl to woman is met by silence in our society. Instead of celebrating, women fear for their daughters, concerned with what kind of girls they will become and what should be said regarding contraception, pregnancy and marriage.

This initial loss is perceptively described by Eichenbaum & Orbach (1985). Little girls are brought up to enact the caring and nurturing role towards others. At the same time they learn to sacrifice their own needs for care and nurturance in the interests of those others and for the majority of women these needs remain unfulfilled. Looking to men to satisfy these needs leaves women bereft, for men have not had the previous learning experiences necessary to the provision of care and nurturance. Eichenbaum & Orbach (1985) point out that such a loss 'causes tremendous pain, confusion, disappointment, rage and guilt for the daughter' but it 'is buried and denied in the culture at large as well as in the unconscious of the little girl'.

A teenager struggling to establish her separate identity and independence may experience loss on two fronts. In the first instance mother, who up and until this time had been cherished and loved unquestionably, is suddenly realised to be just like any other person. This may come as a great shock for both mother and daughter, for mother finds herself frequently under attack while daughter grieves for the lost ideal of the perfect mother. It is part of the maturation process but this knowledge makes it no less difficult.

A second source of loss may occur as the young girl recognises that her form is not flawless; that she is not beautiful and that she appears awkward and graceless. If society were not so remorseless in the pursuit of feminine perfection, women would have less need to feel loss regarding their body image, and perhaps eating disorders like anorexia nervosa would be less common.

Motherhood itself is often touched by loss. When consideration is given to the fact that one in three pregnancies is terminated spontaneously, it is remarkable that so little has been written on the subject; yet only recently have we begun to document and explore the loss that these women suffer. Women who desire children but are unable to conceive for physiological reasons also experience great loss. It may shape the entire course of their lives. Here I would say that we have had some success, for the problems of infertility are now well recognised and publicised.

Moving on to the birth of a baby, the question which is almost inevitably asked is 'Is it all right?' We want to know that we have brought a perfect living being into the world. Great is the joy when we are reassured that the infant is perfect and that we are responsible for its perfection. Sadness, desperation, anger, and guilt may accompany the birth of a baby which is less than perfect.

Inherent in a child's development is the movement away from mother and family to the wider community: it is a necessary task of childhood. Mothers know this intellectually: they facilitate a child's growth by encouraging and involving them in activities outside the home. However, growth may be accompanied by loss as a woman comes to terms with her child's ever-increasing independence. Sadness is present as one sees the layers of innocence peeled away; as one observes the child successfully manage the first day of school; as one realises that friends occupy an increasingly significant place in the child's affections. No one is denying that this progress should be impeded, but it is part of motherhood that one gives birth to a child who eventually must depart. And in this sense women experience loss.

With childbearing complete another form of loss is encountered; that of functional loss. Many women now view the cessation of the menstrual cycle as a positive event. They are free from monthly hormonal imbalances and the attending problems, plus the threat of further children. Sexual activity may be enhanced because one is liberated from the fear of pregnancy. On the other hand, some women see the menopause not as a beginning but as an end to their usefulness.

Increasing age seems to come harder for women than men. I have always thought that it seems rather unjust that men as they grow older become grey and distinguished while women become handsome or just grow old. The pursuit of beautification of the female form through cosmetics, dress and shape, make the ageing process inevitably difficult for women.

Retirement also has the potential for loss. As the numbers of working women increase it can be anticipated that they will meet many of the problems men suffer in adapting to a life without regular employment. A housewife may encounter a different set of problems on her husband's retirement. She has spent a lifetime establishing and maintaining a network without her spouse's presence: in one fell swoop he is at home continuously. Unless the man has maintained outside interests removed from work and home, it is likely that the woman will experience a threat to her autonomy and, subsequently, a loss as a man invades what has been her territory.

The experience of loss is an integral part of the human condition. Loss may be profound as with the death of a child, a spouse or a significant person. It may be traumatic in the wake of divorce, separation or illness. Or it may be an accumulation of many incidents throughout a lifetime.

Health-seeking behaviours: coping behaviour

The following section deals with a variety of behaviours and its content has been selected to highlight some of the issues involved from a female perspective.

Depression

Statistically, women are more prone to depression than men. Fischel (in Fogel & Woods, 1981) notes only a few exceptions to this rule. These are:
1 Widowed or single persons have equal rates of depression.
2 Unemployed married men are more depressed than unemployed married women.
3 Women in professional or managerial jobs have low rates of depression.

She also notes that there is no relation between the menopause and depression, or the departure of children from the home and depression, except in those instances where children have been the major focus of a woman's life.

Colloquially, we speak of 'being depressed'. What is probably meant by this expression is that we feel low, down, or 'not on top of it', maybe as the result of family arguments, a shortage of cash, or as part of premenstrual tension. Used in this way, feeling depressed is a response to the normal ups and downs of daily life. Most of us have experienced this type of emotion and know that, given time, it will be resolved and we will feel better.

Grief is felt after the loss of a significant person (i.e. spouse, child, parent, special friend). It may also occur following certain kinds of surgical intervention such as limb amputation or the removal of sexual organs as in mastectomy or hysterectomy.

Loss of a cherished ideal, aspiration or object may also give rise to grief.

Normally, society recognises the pain involved in grief. Rituals, tradition and ceremony allow us to express our grief openly so that the process of healing and learning to live without that important part may begin. Given this, it is especially cruel that parents whose babies die 'in utero' or shortly after birth are refused the right or bury their infants or register them as dead. For these parents there are no rituals to mark the passing of a life.

Depression is qualitatively different from either the 'blues' or the grieving process. The latter two are usually self-limiting and are responses to specific events. Depression, on the other hand, is a more profound state which is characterised by feelings of loss, low self-esteem, worthlessness, shame, guilt or hopelessness. Physical symptoms may accompany the illness: these include loss of appetite, weight loss, poor quality of sleep whereby there is difficulty in either falling asleep or in remaining asleep, loss of interest in sex and life generally, lessening of interest in personal hygiene and dress, and vague complaints of ill-health.

The individual who is depressed may feel overwhelmed by life. She is bound up in private misery and has no energy to expend on others. Any energy present is utilised to keep herself going at whatever level that can be managed. Eventually, if help is not forthcoming, she may view life as simply not living; everything seems futile and she feels hopeless regarding herself and her power to alter the course of life.

A multitude of theories exist to explain causative factors in depression. However, for out purposes two of the models in Table 5.1 are seen to be of particular relevance for women: life stressors and learned helplessness.

Life Stressors Most psychiatrists would accept that a relationship exists between stress and depression. It would also be true to say that while all people undergo stressful life events, not all become depressed.

The women's movement has provided impetus to the theory of stress-derived depression. Stress may be derived from any of the following:
1 Major life events, e.g. death of a spouse or a significant other relative, divorce, separation, marriage.

Table 5.1 Summary of models of causation of sever mood disturbances (Stuart & Sundeen, 1983)

Genetic	Transmission through heredity and family history
Object loss	Separation from loved one and disruption of attachment bond
Aggression turned inward	Turning of angry feelings inward against oneself
Personality organisation	Negative self-concept and low self-esteem influence one's belief system and appraisal of stressors
Cognitive	Hopelessness experienced because of negative cognitive set
Learned helplessness	Belief that one's responses are ineffectual reinforcers in the environment cannot be controlled
Behavioural	Loss of positive reinforcement in life
Biochemical	Impaired monoaminergic neurotransmission
Life stressors	Response to life stress from four possible sources: major life events, roles, coping resources, and physiological changes.
Integrated	Interaction of chemical, experiential, and behavioural variables acting on the diencephalon

2 Roles, e.g. sexual stereotyping of women as wives, mothers or nurturants.
3 Coping resources, e.g. occupation, financial security, status, family network, community resources.
4 Physiologic changes, e.g. physical trauma, drug-induced alterations from prescribed medication, alcohol and drug dependencies.

In looking for confirmation of the relationship between social stressors and depression Ilfeld's (1977) research is helpful. He found in a study of over 2,200 adults that 'stress in the primary adult relationship (i.e. stress of marriage or of being single) is the life area most closely related to depression'. Furthermore, he asserts that 'there is a direct and dramatic relationship between depression and the total number of stressors experienced' by individuals. Ilfeld's (1977) findings are summarized in Table 5.2

Table 5.2 Relationship between current social stressors and depression

	Employed married mothers	Employed married fathers	Unemployed married mothers	Employed single women	Employed single men
Stressors in descending priority	Marriage	Marriage	Marriage	Financial	Singlehood
	Parenthood	Job	Homemaking	Singlehood	Financial
	Financial	Financial	Parenthood		Neighbourhood
	Neighbourhood	Parenthood	Financial		Job
	Job	Neighbourhood	Neighbourhood		
	Homemaking				

It would seem that many women are, for a variety of reasons, unable to articulate the demands that marriage imposes upon them. They may never have thought that marriage itself contributes to stress. Tensions may be disguised as concerns regarding children, their own state of health or their husband's employment status. Dissatisfaction with marriage may be rationalised in tems of perceived personal inadequacies or the need to preserve the family intact.

Ilfeld's research supports the view that marriage is a stressful life event and, as such, could be put forward as an area worthy of professional interest. If this is the case, health professionals need to develop additional skills in assessing stress from marriage itself.

Learned Helplessness Helplessness is the belief that one cannot achieve a desired outcome. It incorporates feelings of lack of influence or control over one's life. As such, helplessness is related to power in that one either does not have power or is unable to exert the power one possesses.

Seligman in Stuart & Sundeen (1983), proposes that it is not loss in itself which produces depression but rather lack of control over significant life events which prevents individuals from making adaptive responses. Three dimensions are proposed to explain the relationship between helplessness and depression, and these are illustrated in Table 5.3

Table 5.3 Factors in learned helplessness

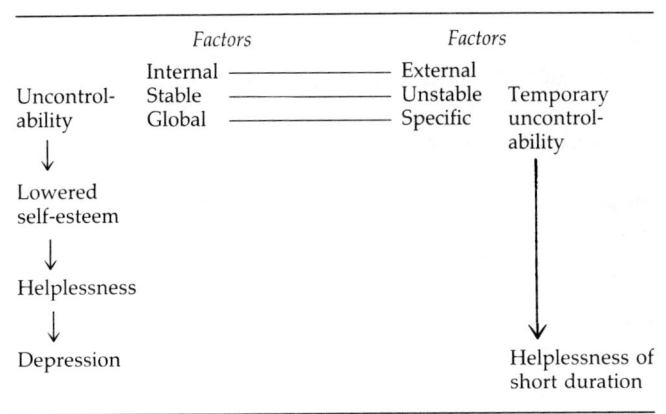

	Factors	Factors	
	Internal ———	External	
Uncontrol-	Stable ———	Unstable	Temporary
ability	Global ———	Specific	uncontrol-ability
↓			↓
Lowered self-esteem			
↓			
Helplessness			
↓			↓
Depression			Helplessness of short duration

The individual who attributes her powerlessness to personal inadequacies (internal factors) is at far greater risk than one who admits lack of control owing to current problems (external factors) such as illness or job loss. The lack of control may be compounded by being a stable feature of one's life; for instance, where one spouse dominates the other. A third complicating factor occurs when the expectation is held that nothing will change in the future (global factors). Thus, helplessness is confirmed by internal belief and lack of control over the foreseeable future and across all situations.

Temporary helplessness, as the term suggests, is a short-lived phenomenon in response to specific situations. It does not involve the lowering of self-esteem, for the causes are seen to lie outside of an individual's personal control.

It is postulated that learned helplessness in women is derived from the internalisation of role expectations. Females are taught from an early age to sublimate their competencies for fear of appearing aggressive or threatening to male aspirations: thus, young girls are socialized into helplessness.

As a variant of this theme, Robinowitz *et al.* (1981) point out that 'women are apt to fail not only because of lack of experience with success but because they themselves have conflicts about success. When a man is successful his manliness is enhanced, but when a woman is successful her feminity is in question'.

When this pattern of female development is considered next to the higher rates of depression reported by married women, the argument that sexual stereotyping plays a role in female depression is more easily appreciated.

Dependency

'Dependency needs are a universal aspect of human experience' (Lerner 1983). The struggle to achieve a balance between dependent – interdependent action constitutes a major developmental task for both sexes, yet given the universality of the task, dependency is usually perceived as a female characteristic. Fogel (in Fogel & Woods 1981) reports that research findings on female dependency are inconclusive. The belief that, in comparison to men women are more passive, dependent and more easily influenced, has yet to be confirmed by empirical study.

Lerner (1983), however, states that 'women more frequently

display pathological dependency; such women do not take action to solve their own problems, do not state clearly their opinions and preferences out of fear, of conflict and disapproval, turn fearfully away from the challenges of the outside world, and avoid successful "autonomous functioning at all costs".' She goes on to argue the case that women are seldom as dependent as they appear to be; rather, they have learned to display passive-dependent behaviour in order to protect significant others and maintain a state of equilibrium in which any attempt to be more assertive or independent is regarded as a betrayal or as an aggressive act. This behaviour is seen to be culturally prescribed and reflects traditional female roles.

The message persists that the weaker sex must protect the stronger sex by not allowing the stronger sex to see the strength of the weaker sex so that the stronger sex need not be threatened by the strength of the weaker sex. One needs only engage a group of women conversationally on this subject to determine that the message holds true.

Women learn very quickly and early in their lives that autonomous, self-directed behaviour is viewed as threatening, aggressive and hurtful. Lerner (1983) suggests that female dependent behaviours are 'often an unconscious "gift" or sacrifice to those they love: it is the giving up self so that the other may gain in self'. Of course, men who wished to treat wives as partners and equals would not accede to this sacrifice.

It is interesting to note that few health professionals consider the context of female dependency to be of any import, yet Lerner (1983) puts forward an articulate case for such consideration. She points out that unless the functions and purposes of dependency are recognised and identified, little progress towards changes may be made. Furthermore, a recognition of the potential loss that a woman and others may incur must be faced before setting a course for personal autonomy.

Given this context, Hill's (1970) therapeutic goals for working with passive-dependent women are helpful. He recommends that these women need to learn to express real feelings and ideas, make decisions comfortably, accept pleasureable experiences and, lastly, control panic.

Dependency needs are not exclusively female terrain. Both sexes require these needs to be met but women traditionally have been viewed as the more dependent sex. It would seem that scope for change exists in encouraging men to express their dependency needs more openly, concurrently with women moving towards more self-directed behaviour.

Alcohol dependency Alcoholism may be defined as the presistent or recurrent injection of alcohol such that it interferes with one's physical, social, psychological or economic functioning, and has traditionally been viewed as a problem affecting the male segment of the population. Indeed, the bulk of the literature and research in this area reflects the view that alcoholism is essentially a male behaviour. Fishel (in Fogel & Woods 1981) cautions that any reader of research data on alcoholism should interpret it 'as applicable only to men unless the researcher speaks specifically about women'.

Estimates of the number of female alcoholics are difficult to come by owing to the lack of research data. While fewer women than men drink and the incidence of problem drinking is lower for females than males, nonetheless one fact is clear: women are consuming more alcohol. Evidence for this may be gleaned from Alcoholics Anonymous, who report an increase in female members from a ratio one female to five males to the present level of one in three (McConville 1983).

Part of the difficulty in assessing the true level of female alcoholism arises from the lack of visibility of female alcoholics. Women who drink excessively are less likely to present themselves for treatment because of the greater social stigma attached to female drinking. Criteria for measuring problem drinking reflect male behaviours, and as the patterns for female and male drinking vary considerably there is less likelihood of identifying female alcoholism. Women tend to drink more in their own homes where such behaviour is less noticeable. Furthermore, because many women do not work, or work in a part-time capacity, performance in a job situation is not seen to be deteriorating as would be the case for an employed male alcoholic.

The Royal College of Psychiatrists (1979) states 'that drinking problems among women are on the increase, and one of the prices to be paid for a more equal place for women in society may be their more equal rate of alcoholism'. This cynical statement is not elaborated upon further in the College's report on *Alcohol and Alcoholism* (1979). Rather it is left to Dr Noble,

Director of the National Institute on Alcohol Abuse and Alcoholism (NIAAA) in the U S A, to point out 'that the answer to female alcoholism is not to return women to their former status . . . attempts to limit the life choices of any human being – male or female – can only be detrimental to basic mental health' (in Fogel & Woods, 1981).

Women, like men, drink excessively for a variety of reasons: to relieve tension and anxiety, to feel more comfortable socially, to submerge feelings of inadequacy and loneliness, and to fill a gap in a less than satisfying life. It has been found by Beckman (1978) that the self-esteem of female alcoholics is less than that of male alcoholics or non-alcoholic females.

Sandmaier (in Fogel and Woods, 1981), suggests that women drink because of dependence on males, depression, sex-role conflicts, specific life crises such as divorce, low self-esteem, anxiety and guilt, conflicts revolving round traditional roles, lack of occupational skills, economic dependency and child-rearing responsibilities which prevent them from entering treatment programmes. In addition, the marketing of alcohol exerts social pressure on women to drink. Alcohol is sold through the images of sex, sand and sun, not on the basis of fetal abnormalities, prostitution or loneliness.

It is essential that research be carried out specifically into female alcoholism. We need more information on how to identify potential high-risk females. We need to know which treatment modalities are best suited to women and their particular problems. There may be certain skills which women need to develop to help them cope more satisfactorily and thus decrease the likelihood of alcohol abuse.

Preventive mental health strategies: skill training

This last section is not intended to be prescriptive in nature for this would indicate that there is a 'right' way of achieving mental health. Rather, the measures mentioned are seen as possible ways forward, some of which may be appropriate for some women.

Primary prevention is aimed at influencing predisposing factors, identifying and assessing precipitating stressors and recognising coping strategies and resources. Primary prevention is usually promoted through the following: health education, environmental change and support from the social system. Health education involves information-giving, and teaching-learning strategies. As such, it may be used to provide and/or strengthen specific skills designed to improve overall life competencies. Environmental change is directed at modifying the immediate environment or the social system at large. Finally, social system support incorporates mechanisms for protecting and/or softening the impact of potential or existing crises. Support may be obtained from within the health system or from self-help groups (i.e. Alcoholics Anonymous) or from agencies operating under specific mandates National Society for the Prevention of Cruelty to Children (NSPCC).

The literature on strategies to aid women to achieve an improved level of mental health is almost exclusively North-American. It reflects the greater strides made in presenting and achieving issues of concern to women to the wider public. Cultural differences towards women, politics, and in this case psychiatry, undoubtedly also play a part. It is unlikely that women in the UK would wish to adopt wholeheartedly the strategies employed elsewhere, yet there is much to learn from others' experience and we may want to adapt some of their acquired knowledge while, at the same time, developing mechanisms more suited to our particular situation.

It would seem initially that health professionals need to have their level of consciousness raised concerning the issues that confront women. Education of the health professional must occur on two fronts: firstly, within existing training programmes and, secondly, for those already in post no matter what their location or level. We need to talk to women about themselves, their lives, their aspirations, their perceptions, their values, and we need to share this information with both sexes and the population at large.

Social change can also be promoted on two levels: the microscopic, that is at the level of the individual, and the macro-level wherein a change is manufactured across society. The two approaches can be complementary in that change at the individual level is promoted and supported by existing networks and change at the wider level is enacted through legislation and policy statements.

David (1980) writes 'to accomplish effective change women need, first and foremost, to trust themselves and reclaim authority over themselves and their own experiences'. She advocates a process of change which includes self-validation, an understanding of how women are subjected to psychological pressure, an understanding of the origins of their own behaviour, increased body awareness, the release of internalised painful feelings and specific skill training.

If we consider skill training it is possible to delineate three distinct levels. The first concerns a woman's own sense of self, a personal level, so to speak; the second level is directed at women gaining control externally, or learning to master the environment, and the last is a maintenance level wherein support systems are organised and participated in. Table 5.4 sets out each level with its attending tasks:

Table 5.4 Skill training levels

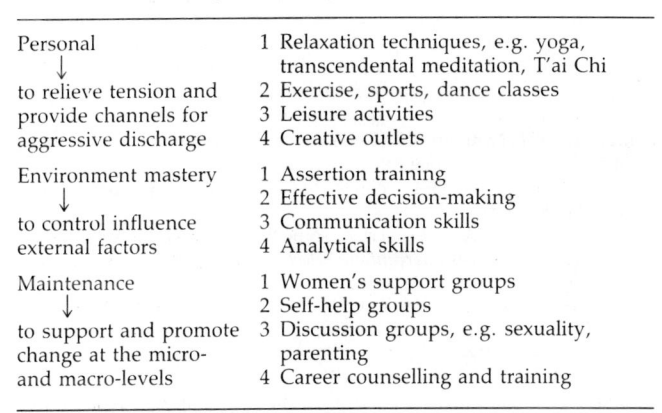

Personal ↓ to relieve tension and provide channels for aggressive discharge	1 Relaxation techniques, e.g. yoga, transcendental meditation, T'ai Chi 2 Exercise, sports, dance classes 3 Leisure activities 4 Creative outlets
Environment mastery ↓ to control influence external factors	1 Assertion training 2 Effective decision-making 3 Communication skills 4 Analytical skills
Maintenance ↓ to support and promote change at the micro- and macro-levels	1 Women's support groups 2 Self-help groups 3 Discussion groups, e.g. sexuality, parenting 4 Career counselling and training

The foregoing provides some indication of how women might be able to proceed in order to facilitate and support change within themselves and the community, but as has been mentioned previously, those who seek to promote change must first appreciate the context and the consequences of any proposed change. Without such understanding, women may simply feel under attack, pressurised, devalued and criticised. As the object is to improve the lot of women let us not do to ourselves what society has done to us from time immemorial.

References

Beckman L J (1978) Self-esteem of women alcoholics. *Journal of Studies in Alcohol*, **39**

Collier P (1982) Health behaviours in women. *Nursing Clinics of North America*, **17**(1)

David S J (1980) Working effectively with women. *Canada's Mental Health*, **28**(2), 2

Editorial (1981) *American Journal of Psychiatry*, **138**(10)

Eichenbaum L & Orbach S (1985) *Understanding Women*. Harmondsworth: Penguin Books

Fogel C I & Woods N F (1981) *Health Care of Women: A Nursing Perspective*. St Louis: C V Mosby Co

Gillis L (1972) *Human Behaviour in Illness*. London: Faber

Hill D (1970) Outpatient management of passive dependent women. *Hospital and Community Psychiatry*, **21**, 402

Ilfeld F (1977) Current social stressors and symptoms of depression. *American Journal of Psychiatry*, **134**(161)

Leickner P & Kalin R (1981) Sex-role ideology among practising psychiatrists and psychiatric residents. *American Journal of Psychiatry*, **138**(10)

Lerner H E (1983) Female dependency in context: some theoretical and technical considerations. *American Journal of Orthopsychiatry*, **53**(4)

McConville B (1983) *Women Under the Influence: Alcohol and its Impact* London: Virago

Nadelson C C & Notman M T (1981) To marry or not to marry. *American Journal of Psychiatry*, **138**(10)

Nairne K & Smith G (1983) *Dealing with Depression*. The Women's Press Handbooks Series

Rapoport L (1965) The state of crisis: some theoretical considerations. In Parrad H J (ed) *Crisis Intervention: Selected Readings*, New York: Family Service Association of America

Robinowitz C B, Nadelson C C & Notman N T (1981) Women in academic psychiatry. *American Journal of Psychiatry*, **138**(10)

Royal College of Psychiatrists (1979) *Alcohol and Alcoholism*. London: Tavistock Publications, London

Stephenson S & Walker G (1979) Mothers – Guilty or Not-Guilty? *Canada's Mental Health*, **27**(1)

Stuart G W & Sundeen S J (1983) *Principles and Practice of Psychiatric Nursing*. St Louis: C V Mosby Co

Trower P, Bryant B & Argyle M (1978) *Social Skills and Mental Health*. London: Methuen

Vincent M O (1981) Marriage and Mental Health *Canda's Mental Health*, **29**(3)

Chapter 6

THE DEVELOPMENT OF WELL WOMAN CLINICS

Pat Thornley

Since the late 1960s and early 1970s, women have become increasingly critical of the type and quality of health care offered to them, as has been discussed in previous chapters. Women began to realise that not only did they need to regain control over their bodies, but that the means of achieving this was through mutual support and self-education which would enable them to develop their self-confidence and a positive attitude to their health so that they could make their needs known to the health professionals. This was to lead to the development of a women's health movement. Groups of women around the country began to campaign for changes in maternity care, gave support to NHS workers resisting cuts in the service and promoted self education and health education. From this positive approach to women's health emerged the concept of well woman clinics which would provide health care more sensitive to women's needs.

British women's health movement

The visit to Britain in 1973 by Carol Downer, a keen advocate of the American self-care movement, provided the initial focus for the formation of a British women and health movement. A number of groups emerged around the country, to promote an awareness of women's health issues by increasing women's knowledge of their own bodies and thus demystifying the medicalisation of their health. There were pressure groups aimed at gaining qualitative improvements in many aspects of health care, such as midwifery (Leeson & Gray 1978).

Within the health movement a fundamental difference on the

approach to the concept of health care emerged between those who sought to divorce themselves from the present system of health care and those who, although recognising its failings, sought changes within the existing framework. Despite this disagreement, it was recognised that there was an overriding necessity for the continuation of women's groups and self-education. Furthermore, the emphasis was to be on the promotion of preventive rather than curative medicine. Whilst acknowledging alternative approaches to the promotion of health, there was a concentration on a practical approach which included issues related to women health workers, health service cuts, radical midwifery and the provision of well woman clinics (Leeson & Gray 1978).

Well woman clinics are intended to provide a service specifically geared to meet the perceived health needs of women. The demand for such clinics has been influenced by the spread of ideas related to early provision of this service in Islington and the perceived inadequacies in existing health care for women. In the North West, women's groups have been particularly interested in this concept and are actively campaigning in various areas for the provision of clinics.

The establishment of the first well woman clinics

It is difficult to trace the actual source of the idea which provided the initial impetus for the campaign and eventual establishment of well woman clinics in Great Britain. It would appear that, at the instigation of community staff, the first clinic was established in February 1973 at Highbury Grange Health Centre, Islington with the aim of expanding the then existing model of health care provided by cervical cytology clinics to provide a more holistic approach to health care, embracing women's physical, social and emotional needs. It was such a success that the fortnightly sessions became weekly, and four more clinics were opened.

During a three-and-a-half-hour session at the clinic ten women are seen, which allows them time to discuss their problems. A health visitor records each woman's medical history and tests her urine and blood pressure. Following this, the doctor carries out breast, abdominal and pelvic examination, takes a cancer smear and swabs, if necessary, and teaches the women self-examination of her breasts. During her time at the clinic, a woman is actively encouraged to discuss any fears or problems that she may have (Roberts 1981).

Treatment is not provided at the clinic and women may attend without referral by their GP. All GPs are notified of their patient's attendance and, if necessary, women are referred back with any problem requiring the GPs attention. Direct referral of women may be made to family planning clinics, special clinics, marriage guidance clinics, social workers and so on.

The clinic provides a much needed service, but does not reach women at risk for cancer screening (Roberts 1981). Hence, take-up of the service is dependent on a woman's motivation. This service has been well publicised since 1977, both locally and nationally, and these ideas provided the catalyst for the demand for well woman clinics in different regions (Islington CHC 1977).

Publicity was achieved through the efforts of women from Islington Trades Council, Essex Road Women's Centre, the National Abortion Campaign and the Community Health Council, and their concern was with the 'high incidence of women with late-discovered cancers (England and Wales and Denmark top the list with the number of cases with breast cancer)' (Islington CHC Annual Report 1976–77).

It was recognised that because of the pressures of family life, women were more likely to ignore their illnesses, particularly at times of high unemployment. The aim was to encourage women to have a positive attitude towards their health. The Area Health Education Department was approached about a campaign to give women health information and advise them on the health screening service at Islington Well Women Clinics. The project was accepted and help and co-operation was offered. Nursing staff at the clinic helped to draft the required publications, which consisted of a poster and five pamphlets providing information on various aspects of women's health. This material formed part of an information pack for display at community activities, and the take-up of this display pack was so good that plans were made to translate these into Greek and Turkish. This basic model of health care for women has been a source of inspiration to others, who have modified or expanded it according to the perceived need of their locality.

Current models of well woman clinics

It is possible to argue that there are three main models of well woman clinics in the United Kingdom – the medical model, the holistic model and the self-help model.

The medical model provides clinics based on the medical perceptions of health developed from the local authority cervical cytology clinics. These clinics offer a medical check up consisting of a full medical history, weight and blood pressure recording, blood tests for anaemia and rubella screening, urine tests, examination of the heart, chest, abdomen and breasts, instruction on self-examination of the breasts, pelvic examination and cervical smear.

Advice may be offered on family planning, and on emotional and sexual relationships, and where necessary, referral is made to the appropriate agency. In general, the policy appears to be that the service offered is provided by an all female staff, consisting of a doctor, health visitor or trained nurse, and a receptionist, but, in some clinics male doctors may also be present. Clinic attendance is by appointment and self-referral. If treatment is required the woman is referred back to her GP or hospital. Ten women may be seen during a two-and-a-half or three-hour session.

Demand for change Women's collective demands for improvement to and expansion of this model of health care relate primarily to qualitative changes. The changes demanded are for better geographical distribution, advertising, and so on and highlight the limitation of this model in its failure to meet women's perception of collective and local community needs. These needs may include testing for sicklecell anaemia; multilingual leaflets; crêche facilities; evening clinics, a less clinical atmosphere and with time for discussion, and so on, the provision of outreach workers to encourage women to attend the clinic, and mobile clinics. The later demands are particularly important to housebound women and those women at risk of cervical cancer who, for a variety of reasons, will not attend the clinic.

Of course, women who attend these clinics are gaining some benefit but increasingly there is a debate within women's health groups to move from this professionally-centred approach to one which will take more account of the perceived needs of women. In addition, the medical orientation may discourage social class IV and V women from attending.

The holistic model is based on the belief that clinics must embrace the woman's physical, social and emotional needs. The model incorporates self-help in its approach and seeks to demystify medicine and treat women as equal participants in their health care. The main impetus for the development of this model stemmed from the ideas of the Islington Well Woman Clinic. This was the philosophy underpinning the Manchester clinics described later in this book.

This model has received much publicity from press and television, stimulating renewed interest in health care geared to women's specific needs. Women's groups and CHC's seeking to persuade their DHA's to establish or improve existing clinics view this model of health care as a desirable objective. Analysis based on user questionnaires and comments from other women suggests that whilst there is a high level of satisfaction, there were criticisms relating to organsational structure which made it impossible to provide medical treatment, particularly for women who had attended for that reason. This may be particularly important for some women who do not wish to be referred to their own GP. Although the feedback draws attention to this curative aspect of women's expectations of the clinic, the problem may not easily be resolved, particularly in view of the 'practical relationship between GP's and well woman clinics' (Manchester Well Woman Clinic Proposal, p 9) and the powers which GP's have to act as gatekeepers to services. The benefits from this model are acknowledged and it has continued to evolve and incorporate aspects of a self-help philosophy.

The self-help model is based primarily on a self-help philosophy which encourages an awareness of how women may adopt a positive attitude to their health and lifestyles through mutual support groups. This is achieved by the promotion of health education and shared knowledge, within an informal, egalitarian, organisational structure. It enables women not only to assume responsibility for their health but also to develop the confidence to make informed choices. In part, this model, although influenced by the ideas from Islington and Manchester, appears to owe its origins to the more radical elements of the women's health movement.

The service provided depends on the perceived needs of women and the resources available for clinic premises, equipment and finance. At the minimum, these may be the provision of a room in a local community centre with access to a telephone, but no direct funding. Other clinics may be more fortunate, being offered more accommodation, equipment and generous donations. Clinic staff are volunteers drawn from all walks of life, some of whom may have a health service background. The clinic offers women a chance to talk over their problems in a relaxed informal atmosphere and provides an informal counselling service offering advice and information on a wider variety of issues.

There may also be provision for health discussion groups, self-help groups and training programmes for new volunteers. Medical examination and cervical smear tests, and so on, may not be available, although information and advice on NHS provision is given.

Limitations This model of health care, although popular, is limited because of the lack of medical provision, particularly if existing health care provision is inadequate. Despite this, some women feel that it is desirable to be divorced from mainstream professional-centred health care. Even if doctors work on a voluntary basis in the clinic there are still problems related to status which make it difficult to implement the self-help ethos of sharing skills and collective action.

There is probably a case for incorporating the self-help model with the holistic model, particularly in areas where women are socially and economically deprived of mainstream health care. While the self-help model may be seen as the best way of providing health education, mutual support and raising women's self esteem the main disadvantage lies in the absence of screening facilities. The amalgamation of these two models may be the answer. There are, however, considerable difficulties in any campaign to set clinics up, particularly in a climate of economic constraints. In addition to resource difficulties, women have problems in determining how and where to put forward their demand to effect change. For many women in the health movement, their work background and links with the health service and community health councils has facilitated campaigns.

Values and beliefs

Underpinning the movement towards the existence of well woman clinics is a conflict between professional power and the demand of women for a different form of health care. The issues raised often centre on women's social and economic inequality. As we have seen there have been successful campaigns but often these have had to be within the constraints of existing medical services. This is best illustrated by the evidence of GP's being not only the gate-keeper to resources within the NHS but also of their 'ownership' of the patient/client.

The debate over health-care provision and gender inequalities must also be seen within the context of class inequalities. Although the need for a united and cohesive women's health movement is recognised, the social divisions within this must be acknowledged. Well woman clinics should be concerned about the quality and value of the service and ensure equal access and provision. The women in greatest need may have the most difficulty in achieving the objectives of a well woman clinic because they first have to overcome the major barriers of racial or class origins, and while the self-help ethos may be seen to be desirable it is necessary to recognise that it may be seen as a useful excuse to cut back services.

Individualism and self-help

The rationale of the present government's approach to health care incorporates 'a tenacious set of market values' and a belief in individualism (Townsend & Davidson 1980, p 33) which may be traced to the Victorian era and the emergence of a philosophy promoting individualism, self-help and minimum State intervention. This philosophy, deriving from the economic rationale of laissez faire and Benthamite utilitarianism, shaped Victorian attitudes to welfare provision and legitimise the State's non-interventionary role. Failure to make provision for oneself and one's dependents was seen as an inherent defect resulting from idle and spendthrift ways. Despite State intervention in the sphere of public health, medical care was characterised primarily by private philanthropy and self-help.

Although by the early 1900s the Liberal government's concern for national efficiency and fear of socialism provided the impetus for the implementation of wide-ranging social policies, nevertheless this collective action was underpinned by the notion of individualism. The limited National Health Insurance, whilst of undoubted benefit, was based, in part, on compulsory employee contributions. Similarly, measures to effect improvement in infant mortality rates were primarily concerned to educate the mothers in the means by which this may be achieved.

This pragmatic approach to welfare provision was reflected in the recommendations of the Beveridge Report. Thus, although Beveridge underlined the need for collectivist strategies in the approach to welfare provision, in effect there was no fundamental change. Despite incorporating the notions of collectivism and universalism, he retained the principle of individualism, enshrining it in compulsory social insurance (Fraser 1973, p 200). It was a pragmatic response to the limited nature of welfare provision and fitted current notions of what future provision should be. In effect, it sought to balance the needs of labour and capital in a planned and rational manner.

Although the concept of individualism did not appear to be the dominant principle in the emergence of the welfare state, it characterised the individualistic approach to health within the NHS. However, it may be suggested that in times of economic recession individualism appears to return to its former position of dominance. From the mid 1970s the emphasis on individualism has grown, particularly in relation to health care. Although there has been a shift in emphasis from curative to preventive medicine, it is within the context of individual responsibility. This emphasis on the need for a healthier lifestyle diverts attention from the social and economic environmental factors contributing to ill health.

Despite evidence of major cutbacks in public expenditure and future proposed cutbacks, particularly in the NHS, the Conservative Government under Mrs Thatcher was returned to office in 1983. Protests over reductions in expenditure on the NHS, education and so on remain localised and sporadic. This begs the question of how, despite an apparent collective commitment to the welfare state, the government is able to legitimise its social and economic policies. These underline the contraditions inherent within the State's role of legitimisation and accumulation. However, perhaps Mrs Thatcher's apparent strength lies in her perceptiveness in resurrecting the notion of individualism and the norms and values underpinning this. By appealing to the needs for individual and collective sacrifices to achieve economic recovery, the notion of individualism legitimates cutbacks in public expenditure and the privatisation necessary for capital accumulation (Hall & Jaques 1983, p 301).

This emphasis on individualism and self-help poses a double threat to women. The self-help philosophy and the goals and values underpinning it must be made explicit as they could dovetail with Thatcherite notions of self-help and proposed cutbacks. Women's previous historic gains have reflected this duality, in that apparent gains by women, in effect, serve the interests of patriarchy and capitalism. Hence, reforms in working condition, although protecting women from long hours and hazardous occupations, effectively reduced female competition for jobs. Likewise, return to the home ensured the continued production and reproduction of a healthy workforce.

The Education Act 1944, despite offering equal opportunities to all, reinforces the stereotyping of male and female roles in relation to the socio-economic structure. Women's expectations, particularly those created through access to further education, are not realised in the economic reality of the labour market, and opportunities may be restricted on the basis of their reproductive role.

The well woman clinics, particularly those based on voluntarism and collective self-help, may fit the present economic policies. Nevertheless, they also represent a fundamental shift in the orientation of attitudes to health and health-care delivery. In seeking to challenge the medical expert's role they challenge the patriarchal base of the social relationships contained within a capitalist system of health care, although further research is required to examine its long-term effects.

References

Community Health Council News (1978) *Well Woman Clinic.* 27(1), 10
Fraser D (1973) *The Evolution of the British Welfare State.* London Monthly Review Press

Hall S & Jaques M (eds) (1983) *The Politics of Thatcherism*. Oxford University Press

Islington Community Health Council *Annual Report 1976/77*. Manor Gardens Centre, 6/9 Manor Gardens, London N7 6LA

Leeson J & Gray J (1978) *Woman and Medicine*. London: Tavistock Publications

Roberts H (ed) (1981) *Women, Health and Reproduction*. London: Routledge & Kegan Paul

Townsend P & Davidson N (eds) (1982) *Inequalities in Health*. Harmondsworth: Penguin Books

Chapter 7

THE MANCHESTER EXPERIENCE I: WYTHENSHAWE WELL WOMAN CLINIC

Rebekah Williams

Background

There are two well woman clinics in South Manchester, known collectively as The South Manchester Well Woman Clinics. The main aim of this chapter is to define what is meant by a well woman clinic, and to give an account, from a lay worker's perspective, of why and how the first such clinic in the North West came into the being. In the next chapter Joan Armstrong will describe how these clinics work in practice, and how some health professionals, like herself, came to see well woman clinics as fitting into their role both as women and as professional workers in the primary and preventive health service.

Wythenshawe Well Woman Clinic was established in July 1981 and is perhaps the most famous of its kind. Its opening attracted a great deal of positive publicity on television, radio and the local and national press. As a consequence, it was not long before it was seen by many women's health groups as a model of the sort of service that they would like to see available in their own communities.

Well woman clinic campaign groups now exist in approximately 50 areas throughout the United Kingdom, and at some time have either visited our clinics, requested information from us and/or have invited us to speak at their local public meetings. In our experience these groups are predominantly organised by volunteers who have little or no professional training as health workers, and who are constantly frustrated by the lack of interest in or any apparent understanding of the concept of a well woman clinic by their respective health authorities and professional health workers. More often than not the groups come up against arguments that the services being asked for already exist, or that by simply adding a new title of 'Well Woman Clinic' to services such as the Family Planning and Cytology Clinics, the groups' demands will be met. By documenting the series of events and the basic philosophy that led to the establishment of our well woman clinics, and our current position, it is hoped to dispel these misconceptions and to argue that well woman clinics are a necessary future feature of a National Health Service which has long been criticised for failing adequately to meet women's needs (Illich 1975; Newman 1984).

In an attempt to bridge the gap between women's needs and the services offered, women began to create alternative services. The development of organisations such as the National Childbirth Trust (1956), the British Pregnancy Advisory Service (1968), the Brooke Advisory Centres (1964) and the Women's National Cancer Control Campaign (1965), gave early signs that women were prepared, if necessary, actually to plan and implement certain aspects of their health care outside the NHS.

Contrary to popular opinion the current pressure being placed upon the medical profession to relinquish their control over women's bodies is not new. What is different today is that the women's health movement has changed in important ways that invest it with the potential for bringing about lasting change in how women's health needs are perceived and dealt with.

In the late 1970s and early 1980s local women's groups around the country began to set up informal Women and Health Discussion Courses where various common womens' health problems were dealt with from a non-medical perspective. These proved to be extremely popular, attracting large numbers of women who were keen to take up an opportunity to learn about their health and, in particular, to find alternative methods of coping with or eliminating certain problems from their lives. Out of these courses it emerged that women were disillusioned with a male-dominated medical profession that generally dismisses trivia problems such as period pains, menopausal problems, vaginal discharges, thrush, cystitis and sexual and other relationship difficulties.

In short, the action taken by small groups of women in the community offered what had previously been lacking – an opportunity for women to gain an in-depth understanding of their specific health needs and to collate and disseminate self-help knowledge on how to tackle them. In addition, they facilitated the rapid growth of a movement where women, irrespective of age, culture, status, religion, social class, sexual orientation and of feminist or non-feminist tendencies, could collectively voice what many had felt individually. Today's women's health movement is one which has culminated in a demand for radical change in attitudes to health care, away from the disease-orientated domain of the doctor to a holistic, preventive approach, reflecting the diverse needs of its major consumer – women.

The movement continues to thrive both locally and nationally, and to be fed by initiatives outside the NHS. Television programmes and magazine articles on women's health issues are now commonplace, women and heath courses continue to be popular and have now been adopted financially by organisations such as The Workers' Education Association. Community workers have also been appointed by some local authorities who among other activities run health projects specifically designed for women. The well woman clinics' campaigns play an important and integral part in the womens health movement, and the birth of the Wythenshawe Clinic was seen as a major breakthrough for the movement as a whole.

Joan Armstrong explains later that an important feature of the current movement is the increasing number of community-based health professionals who find that traditional approaches to health care may be obstructive to their efforts to provide effective preventive health programmes. It would be unjust not to acknowledge and congratulate those individuals within the health profession who had already successfully attempted to implement changes of practice in line with those being voiced by women's health movements. By the late 1970s some GPs in Liverpool, Salford, Western Super Mare, Birmingham, High Wycombe and Nottingham had organised a well woman session within their practices and in Islington and Leicestershire health areas health visitors and community medical officers had established well woman sessions in five and eight health centres respectively. However, it was not until the creation of the Wythenshawe Well Woman Clinic that lay women were 'allowed' to participate in the planning and implementation of a completely new service within the NHS.

There were three basic ingredients in the recipe that eventually produced the Wythenshawe Clinic: an active women's group, situated in Levenshulme in the Central District, sympathetic and supportive CHCs in all three Districts, and active support by influential women employees, mainly from within South District.

Early days at Wythenshawe: the first year

The Clinic was opened in July, 1981, and as with all new projects it was expected that teething problems would occur. The financial constraints imposed on the Clinic however, led to the creation of additional unforeseen problems.

In the well woman clinic proposals several references were made to the fact that the pilot Clinic should be seen as being experimental in nature, and that as such the venture would need to be flexible and open to change and development in line with the wishes of its workers and clients. There were, however, some fundamental characteristics considered to be central to the purpose and philosophy of a well woman clinic, namely a particular type of clinic structure and a particular team of staff.

The purpose of the well woman clinic as defined in the proposals was:

(a) 'to reach women who normally stay away from doctors for reasons of class, culture or because they are intimidated by male GPs;

(b) to try to find effective ways of meeting women's specific health problems;

(c) to develop a general understanding about health care provision and the obstacles to improvement both within the medical profession and in the community, so that services and information which will contribute to the good health of an individual and the community can be offered and accepted.'

The main target group of the clinic was defined at the outset as 'women who rarely, if ever, visit their doctor and who are believed medically to be most at risk, ie. the disadvantaged, the poor, the infertile and the older women'.

In order to achieve the clinic's purpose and to attract its target group the proposals set out details of three types of session: the clinic session, the discussion group and the self-help group – these are described in the next chapter.

Having detailed the type of service that was to be offered, the proposals then discussed who would provide that service: according to the proposals the simplest and most effective group of staff included the following personnel: community development worker, health education worker, health visitor, doctor, social worker and crêche worker. The community development worker was seen as the only full-time member of the Well Woman Clinic staff: her role would be to co-ordinate the services offered and present them to the public. She would be responsible for the organisation and administration of the Clinic as well as actually participating in the three types of clinic sessions.

The roles that each of the other members of the well woman team was expected to develop were clearly linked to their training and usual professional activities. The proposals envisaged that although all the basic medical and counselling services would be provided by paid employess of the NHS or the local authority, local volunteer workers would be encouraged to work with the professionals. Their contribution to the team was seen to be important in establishing a vital link between the Clinic and the community. It was suggested that the volunteers could act in a watch-dog capacity to ensure that the aims and philosophy behind the setting up of the Clinic were adhered to. The proposals stated, however, that the service offered should not be dependent upon voluntary help as this is 'often unreliable and usually takes more time to organise than the help it provides'. Overall, the general theme underlying the staffing section of the proposals was that a committed and harmonious well woman team was a prerequisite for the success of the entire venture.

The task of the Clinic organiser (principally the Specialist in Community Medicine, South District) was to produce the above components of a well woman clinic at no additional cost. This she proceeded to do by the only option open to her – the juggling and redistribution of resources already available.

Implementing the proposals

The main consequence of having no extra monies was that the idea of employing a full-time clinic worker to co-ordinate the project was no longer practicable. This inevitably meant that all administration had to be undertaken from the office of the Specialist in Community Medicine: she and her secretaries were now to be the central figures in the organisation of the Clinic. All things considered, the decision to locate the Clinic in South Manchester was, in fact, the only sensible and practical solution.

Accommodation for the Well Woman Clinic was found by establishing where time and space were available in community health centres. As a result, the Clinic was based in the Woodhouse Park Combined Health Centre situated in the heart of the largest council housing estate in Europe, Wythenshawe. This setting and the accommodation were considered to be highly suitable, including as it did a fully-equipped doctor's room. It was, however, available only on a Tuesday afternoon and the Well Woman Clinic could thus only open for one two-hour clinic session per week, instead of the three originally proposed.

Women who were interested and employed in the local community health services were encouraged to make arrangements to work at the Clinic as part of their official jobs. This presented little difficulty for the doctors as their workload was administered by the District Community Physician who had been a keen supporter of the idea from the start. The cost of doctor sessions was thus re-directed to the Clinic from other facilities that had already been cut or were under-utilised. Finding the other staff turned out to be much more of a problem.

All attempts to encourage local health service employees to work at the Clinic were unsuccessful and, with the exception of a community worker from Social Services, active participation or support from other local workers failed to materialise. Consequently, for the Clinic to be able to function at all the organisers had to rely on a workforce that consisted predominantly of women who had been active in campaigning for it. Apart from containing a number of women with a nursing background, this resource also produced a group who were trained in a number of relevant non-clinical skills. These women either agreed to work voluntarily for the Clinic or were in jobs that allowed them sufficient control to choose to work at the Clinic, ie. staff from Manchester University Department of Nursing, health education officials, community workers, psychologists and unwaged women. The Clinic thus got under way with a team of highly motivated staff, with the majority of its members being well versed in the philosophy behind the project, and possessing a pretty clear understanding of how the Clinic was to function. The Well Woman Clinic soon began to offer a service that resembled the one originally envisaged in the proposals. The Tuesday-afternoon Clinic, however, was now staffed by three doctors (two with gynaecological experience and one with a psychiatric background) and an average of two volunteer nurses. In addition, between five and eight lay volunteers attended each session. Clinical duties remained the responsibility of the clinical staff, leaving the other volunteers to carry out the interviewing, look after children, attend to women in the waiting room and deal with problems that did not require a specific medical or nursing input. Clerical duties directly concerned with the session were taken on by a sympathetic clerk who already worked in the Clinic building, a service for which she was soon to be paid by the Health Authority.

All workers were encouraged to attend Policy Meetings where problems and suggestions concerning the Clinic could be raised and discussed. One of the first policy decisions was to design a feedback questionnaire as a means of discovering how women felt about the service. Women attending the Clinic were subsequently asked to fill in the questionnaire and return it in a pre-paid envelope two weeks after their visit. It was envisaged that information received in this way could play an important part in future policy decisions. A new Health Profile Questionnaire was also designed – see Appendix.

Public response to the opening of the Clinic was, to say the least, overwhelming. Volunteers from the original campaign group had been 'bused' into Wythenshawe to conduct a door-to-door leafleting exercise, and posters announcing the Clinic were displayed in prominent public places. At first, the Clinic was attended by a steady trickle of local women. Before long, workers found they were not only dealing with an increasing number of Wythenshawe women who had heard about the Clinic through word of mouth, but also with a substantial number of women from all over the Greater Manchester area. Local and national press, radio and television publicity stimulated interest to such an extent that it was not uncommon to have between 20 and 30 women attending a single session, not to mention countless telephone calls!

Such pressure of numbers presented us with organisational difficulties and unfortunately led to a situation where some outside observers concluded that the Clinic was functioning in a state of 'semi-ordered chaos': we soon found ourselves having to make a major change in Clinic policy.

According to the feedback questionnaires, women who were otherwise satisfied with the service invariably mentioned that they had had to wait for too long before being seen. There was also growing concern among the workers that overcrowded conditions were not condusive to giving the time and attention that were essential ingredients of the Clinic. A policy decision was therefore taken to devise an appointment system for all women living outside Wythenshawe. This decision was not taken lightly, as we were aware that part of the attraction of the Clinic was that women could decide to come and act upon that decision immediately. A three-to-six-week wait for an appointment would inevitably kill that spontaneity. The partial appointment system helped but demand continued to be high, and after several months of running the Clinic with a waiting list of eight weeks and beyond, a further policy decision became necessary. A full appointment system was introduced in April 1982, which restricted clients to residents of the South Manchester District.

Apart from considering how to cope with the pressure of numbers, policy discussion also centred on whether Clinic practice reflected the philosophy of the Clinic. In particular, there was concern that the Clinic structure and the division of duties according to professional labels was inconsistent with our aims of demystifying health care and working in a non-hierarchial way. For most workers the experience of working at the Clinic was seen as a learning exercise where non-medical staff could extend their knowledge of medical aspects of health, and medically-trained workers could, in turn, gain from the knowledge and experience of the other workers. And although it was never seen to be necessary or desirable for all workers to have all the skills used at the Clinic, it was vital that each should be fully aware of what other workers could do to maximise individual resources.

In order to encourage a collective way of working and to facilitate skill sharing and demystification it was decided that workers would not use their professional labels, if any, and would take it in turns to share duties such as looking after women in the waiting area, doing the interviews, looking after children, making the tea, setting up and clearing away the Clinic: thus, it was hoped that communication barriers would be broken down. The exceptions to this rule were the doctors, as no-one else could be expected to carry out their clinical duties. Nevertheless, they too were expected to take an equal share in the rest of the duties when their clinical skills were not in demand, and to share information and decisions with the other workers. The doctors did not wear white coats and although they used their room while examining the women they made regular appearances in the waiting room and shared tea and conversation with everyone else.

After a while, policy meetings began to address ways by which the Clinic could improve its response to the needs that were being expressed by the women attending. Many presented initially as wanting help with common physical female complaints such as thrush, cystitis, and menstrual or menopausal problems, but as the visit progressed it was not unusual to find that they also talked about how their health was affected by their life situation: many mentioned that they were depressed, isolated and bored. In addition, many women said that they lacked the confidence and opportunities to find solutions, especially as most of them had neither training nor skills which were readily marketable. Older women often expressed disappointment and disillusionment with their marriages.

Women came to the Clinic because they had not found effective treatment or sufficient support or information elsewhere. They saw the Clinic as a possible source of sympathetic help from women workers and were attracted by the Clinic's offer of time to talk in a relaxed and informal atmosphere. The majority, however, felt that they needed to suffer physical symptoms in order to justify a visit.

Our experience had shown that it was relatively easy to fulfil expectations of a medical service because performing routine tests is a demand that is easily satisfied. Thanks to the Clinic structure, however, the worker could also explain and promote a positive approach to health. The questionnaire was specifically designed to enable the worker to explain what was being offered and why, and to open up discussion on the advantages of self-help remedies, healthy eating, exercise, breast examination and cervical cytology. The one-to-one interview also gave ample opportunities for women to raise and talk-through aspects of their lives that were affecting their sense of well-being.

For some women, reassurance gained from a medical check-up, together with information received on the various options available to them for dealing with specific health problems, was sufficient for them to think that the time had been well spent. For the majority of others the Clinic visit served as their first opportunity to identify and discuss particular problems, and as a starting point from which to work towards finding solutions. In such instances workers found that time during the Clinic session was being spent simply on building women's confidence in what they already knew about their health and on demystifying health care. Workers increasingly became aware that these women found considerable relief in discovering that they were not alone in their worries and that others were facing similar problems and asking similar questions. As a result, Clinic workers soon recognised the need to offer follow-up activities in the form of self-help groups and discussion courses.

With the help of the Workers Education Association, the volunteers set up weekly discussion courses, open to anyone who wished to attend, on subjects ranging from premenstrual tension, to healthy eating, to the menopause. Attendance at the courses was high but, in particular, they attracted women who were either suffering from stress and anxiety, or who were in their forties or fifties and having difficulty in coping with, or understanding, the physical and/or psychological symptoms of the menopause. A need for two specific groups was thus identified and the workers established a menopause group and a relaxation course.

The Evaluation document

At the end of the first six months the AHA (now DHA) requested that a report be submitted to enable them to ascertain whether the pilot Clinic was achieving its aims. Clinic workers, together with researchers from the Department of Epidemiology and Social Research, carried out an evaluation of the Clinic using two sources of information, namely, the Health Profile Questionnaires completed during the Clinic sessions and the Feedback Questionnaires. As the following quotation illustrates, the results of the exercise, produced in March 1982, were encouraging and left little doubt as to the success of the Clinic thus far.

> 'Overall, the results show that the Clinic fulfilled the aims it set out to achieve. Indeed, from these findings the extent to which the working of the Clinic follows the original objectives is remarkable.
>
> The women who attend reported a large number of difficulties ranging over a wide range of problem areas, being specifically female complaints, and psychological, physical or social problems. The Clinic was used mainly by older women. Virtually no-one used the Clinic simply for screening or a check-up, but all attenders welcomed the opportunity to take advantage of these facilities and most especially welcomed being able to talk over their problems in a relaxed and friendly atmosphere.'
>
> Evaluation of Manchester Well Woman Clinics 1982

The evaluation also confirmed that demand far outstripped original expectations and that the Clinic did appear to fill an important gap in current NHS provision.

At this stage the Well Woman Clinic project seemed to have survived the negative effects of funding problems, and overcome the disappointment that ensued with the realisation that there was little support, and no response, from health workers in the Wythenshawe area. Evidence contained in the evaluation clearly put forward a case for positively encouraging and maintaining a staff comprised of lay and professional people. Formal training in clinical and nursing skills were invaluable to the success of the Clinic, but so too were the skills and personal qualities such as empathy, sensitivity, the ability to listen, communicate and work informally, and these can be found and developed in people from all walks of life.

The Clinic functioned efficiently for the best part of the first year without any formal system of ensuring that particular volunteers signed up for specific sessions. During this time volunteers were numerous and it was possible to practise adequate numbers of staff in coping with busy Clinic sessions. Attempts to organise a definite rota failed because many volunteers were involved in other jobs and could not guarantee specific attendance. In the rare event of there being an insufficient number of volunteers at any one session, a back-up list of women who could stand in at short notice was used.

The problems of erratic staffing levels first emerged when it was discovered that fewer and fewer women were able to continue to give so much of their time to the Clinic because of other commitments. Many of the volunteers came from the original campaign groups in other areas and had always seen their roles in the Wythenshawe Clinic as temporary. Wythenshawe was seen as a breakthrough in that a Clinic had come into being, but for those women it was never seen as an answer to their own communities' demands for such a service. In line with the belief that each well woman clinic should be run according to the wishes of its local female population, Clinic policy had always been to encourage local women to become involved. Women who attended the Clinic were invited to join in policy meetings and either make their opinions and suggestions known and/or offer their services in whatever capacity they felt able. In anticipation of the inevitable slimming down of the original workforce it was hoped that sufficient numbers of new recruits would also emerge through this process and so maintain a consistantly high level of committed volunteers – be they professional or lay.

As it happened, very few Wythenshawe women came forward, and those who did could not be persuaded to try their hand at anything other than helping with the tea. Such offers were welcomed and accepted but they were disappointing. Clinic sessions had highlighted the fact that these women lacked confidence in their own abilities, but despite our efforts to appear otherwise we suspected that we were still probably coming across as offering something that they could not. However, new volunteers from outlying districts did appear and proved to be of great value to the Clinic for three main reasons. Firstly, they included a number of older women with an interest in the menopause; secondly, they were committed to a holistic approach to health; and thirdly, they were in situations where they were ready and able to devote much time and energy to becoming a united team of key workers. Eventually, the Clinic was staffed by a team of two doctors and nine regular volunteers who organised a rota to ensure that a minimum of five volunteers were available each week. In addition, approximately seven other volunteers continued to attend as and when they could. This team soon found itself facing an additional change of staff, which, although not fully realised at the time, would lead to a dramatic change in their circumstances. In April 1982 the NHS was reorganised for the second time in ten years. The main aim of the exercise was to eliminate the Area level of administration and thereby reduce NHS manpower expenditure. Before its demise the AHA considered the results of the Clinic Evaluation they had commissioned and, having expressed satisfaction with the report, endorsed it and duly recommended it to the incoming District Health Authority.

Following the 1982 NHS reorganization, the District Medical Officer and the Specialist in Community Medicine, who had been so supportive, successfully applied for posts elsewhere.

In theory, our endeavours to work collectively and share decision-making, tasks and knowledge, should have protected us against the effects of loosing one member of staff. In practice, however, it emerged that we were ignorant of many things and saying goodbye to our Specialist in Community Medicine in fact amounted to losing our only source of direct administrative, organizational and secretarial contact with the Health Authority. She, above all, understood the potential difficulties that her move could create for us, and, in an attempt to reduce the effects, made a formal recommendation to the Health Authority that a full-time, paid, co-ordinator be appointed to look after the interests of the present Well Women Clinic as well as any future Clinics that may open in the district.

The Search for recognition

Encouraged by the prospect of having a co-ordinator, workers set about organising themselves as best they could. Policy meetings now began to be dominated by administrative and secretarial matters, as well as organisational problems associated with staffing rotas, Clinic sessions, the self-help group and discussion courses.

For their part the volunteers were being placed under more and more pressure, and for a few of the more established volunteers in particular, a good deal of their working week and spare time was spent on well women business. By the end of the first year volunteering at the Clinic entailed not only participating in practically every session and policy meeting, but also participating in activities such as the taking of policy meeting minutes, dealing with a growing number of letters requesting help from women all over the United Kingdom and other correspondence concerning the Clinic, addressing meetings and giving talks on the work of the Clinic both locally and nationally, and organising, welcoming and attending to visitors and potential volunteers who expressed interest in the Clinic.

To make matters worse, we found ourselves suffering from an acute lack of knowledge about where to go for supplies, or who to contact about obtaining further copies of the clinic questionnaire, and so on and so on. Some problems were easily solved, and, as far as she was able from her new position in North District, the Specialist in Community Medicine continued to offer support and information on who to contact for help. Other problems, however, proved more difficult to solve, and before long the cost and labour of servicing the Clinic was, with the exception of postage, met by volunteers themselves or by willing agencies such as Health Education and Community Health Councils in Manchester and elsewhere. Slowly the realisation dawned that many of the administrative staff of the new Health Authority were unaware of our existance or were unsure of how to deal with the clinic or its queries and requests. Morale fluctuated but sufficient good news usually managed to arrive in time to restore our faith in what we were trying to achieve.

On the whole, the period immediately following reorganisation was a difficult time for Clinic workers. The Clinic sessions continued to operate effeciently and apparently to good effect, but the workload required to ensure that this remained so was such that there was little time and energy left for other activities. In effect, the combination of a reduced volunteer staff and increased administrative chores resulted in closure of the discussion and relaxation courses. Staff were also at a loss to see how other forms of necessary outreach work could be carried out in the community, and were aware that without this, local participation in the Clinic was unlikely to happen.

The apparent failure to win acceptance from other health workers also led to questioning how realistic it was to believe that some change in traditional health care attitudes within the Health Service could be brought about. It had always been recognised that of all the aims, this would be the most difficult to achieve. There was a general consensus that it was now of primary importance to concentrate on increasing our workforce by finding a way of developing more interest from Health Service staff and in order to achieve this it was important first to discover why the Clinic produced such a negative response in other health workers.

We were aware that local health workers, in particular, had felt that there had been insufficient consultation with them before the Clinic was set up in their area, and that to some extent we were still bearing the brunt of their disappointment of that time. In an attempt to repair this earlier mistake, invitations to policy meetings and Clinic sessions were extended to health workers in the area: the results, however, highlighted other more fundamental reasons for their wish to remain at a distance. Our way of working, and our use of volunteers in particular, created difficulties and led to the following interpretations of the aims and philosophy of the Clinic. Working with volunteers on an equal basis was construed by some as an exercise in negating their professional skills and training, and our aim to re-educate women to be more assertive when discussing their health care was seen as evidence of our intention to encourage a vote of no-confidence in the health profession. Our holistic approach to health which acknowledged the contribution that environmental and situational factors make to health suggested that the Clinics were political in nature and this, together with the connotations that could be attached to a women-only Clinic, was distasteful to some health professionals.

It seemed that an additional area of difficulty for some health workers related to the conditions of service that apply within the Health Service. Staff are employed for a specific number of hours, and any extra hours spent on work or training is given on the understanding that the time will be repaid to them in kind. The effeciency of the Well Woman Clinic depends upon the development of a teamwork approach and to achieve this it is necessary for its workers to meet outside official Clinic hours. The structure of the Clinic session is also such that the workers find it unusual to finish their work within the two hours allocated. It was made clear to us that unless we could arrange for the repayment of any extra time that the health workers gave, then there would be little hope in expecting many of them to agree to participate.

Given the above it is not difficult to understand that the Well Woman team felt somewhat dispondent about the prospect of finding suitably sympathetic health workers. It seemed that the majority of health workers we had made contact with wished to change and control rather than to help or join the team, and that 'help' in this way entailed thinking which was antagonistic to the philosophy and policy of the Clinic. We strongly suspected, however, that it was the volunteer element which created the problems more than anything else. Health Service workers are unaccustomed to dealing with volunteers and to expect them to be responsive to the requests and ideas of a group who, to all intents and purposes were running an unconventional service, was too much to ask. We felt that the situation would change dramatically if a paid co-ordinator for the Clinic could be appointed by the Health Authority. Such a person would not only be able to relieve the volunteers of their administrative headaches but also have the necessary time, status and skills to work with the health professionals to define more clearly and work through the various obstacles to their involvement in the Clinic.

In August 1982 representatives from the Clinic contacted Health Authority officials and several meetings subsequently took place. At the first meeting a representative from the Clinic explained our administrative difficulties and the reasons why we wished the Health Authority seriously to consider the appointment of a paid Well Woman Co-ordinator. We were informed that reorganisation was still not complete and that the Health Authority's financial position was poor, but they would do what they could to help. Later meetings managed to iron out minor problems such as our mailing and stationery needs, but despite various verbal suggestions that our problems over a co-ordinator would be solved in the near future, nothing concrete occurred.

The tone of the meetings, however, gave us some cause for concern. We got the distinct impression that we were not taken altogether seriously, and we were certain that our status as volunteers meant that we were treated with less respect than was usually shown to Health Authority employees. Eventually the Authority admitted that they knew very little about us and after visiting the Clinic asked that we produce a report.

However, prior to this request, unsatisfactory contact with the Health Authority had prompted us to get in touch with the three health visitors who had established their own Well Woman Clinic in Withington in June 1982. Apart from being attracted by the possible advantage that safety in numbers might procure, we were curious to find out whether they were suffering from similar problems.

This proved to be the most constructive action we had taken since reorganization. Not only did we discover that our Clinics were similar in structure, but also that the staff unreservedly shared our views on the value of a teamwork approach using lay and professional women. It also emerged that although they had fewer administrative, secretarial and organizational problems, they felt the need for a co-ordinator.

A decision to become united officially under the title of 'The South Manchester Well Woman Clinic' was unanimously welcomed by both sets of Clinic staff. So, too, was the suggestion that we organise joint in-service training courses and study days for the benefit of all the workers. In this way it was hoped to facilitate the interchange of information and skills between the workers, and also enable us to meet each other informally away from the pressures of our Clinic sessions in order to establish a better system of mutual support. Together we also designed a training course for new workers and produced our first official Policy Document.

The Wythenshawe Clinic submitted its report to the Health Authority in September 1982 and, as requested, it addressed issues pertinent to our Clinic. Reference was made frequently to the shared needs of the two South Manchester Clinics, and the section dealing with the proposal and job description for a co-ordinator was submitted as a joint request.

After receiving the report the Health Authority began to produce some real solutions to our problems, although it was made plain to us that in a climate of financial constraints it was extremely unlikely that our request for a new Health Authority appointment would be fulfilled.

Community Services secretarial staff undertook to do our typing and mailing and arranged for the reprinting and delivery of our questionnaires by the Regional Health Authority. In addition, we learnt that all volunteers were now going to be paid their travel expenses and that money from Community Services would be made available for us to purchase the books we required for the Clinic library.

At Wythenshawe in particular, we now felt that we were at last achieving some sort of recognition, and morale was considerably boosted. Some degree of integration within the primary and preventive services seemed to be occurring. Wythenshawe now had access to the same services that had always been available to the Withington Clinic and the September report resulted in some encouraging news for the volunteers in both Clinics. These developments, however, did little to change the situation as far as the need for a co-ordinator was concerned and this issue, together with how to encourage more input from Health Service and volunteer staff, continued to dominate discussion for the following year.

When negotiations for a co-ordinator appeared to be getting nowhere the Clinics began to look for alternative sources of funding for such a post. We soon discovered, however, that because we were part of statutory body (NHS), any application would need to come from the Health Authority itself. For their part the Health Authority were reluctant to pursue our suggestion on the grounds that most alternative funding would only cover the cost of a post for a limited period of time, and they would probably still not be in a position to appoint a co-ordinator once that funding had ceased. Instead, it emerged that the Health Authority were hoping to solve the problem by involving more Health Service employees in the work of the Clinic.

Almost one year after the Wythenshawe report the Clinics were informed that a Nursing Officer post for health visiting in Wythenshawe had become vacant. The Management proposed that, if we were willing, the post could be advertised as having an additional special responsibility for the Well Woman Clinics in South Manchester. We were also informed that the Authority intended to upgrade a clerical worker from the Community Services offices to help us with our administrative chores. Both Clinics supported these proposals and although we were aware that the people appointed would find it difficult to do two jobs at once, we were happy to accept the offer.

The arrival of our Nursing Officer and clerical support considerably eased the burden upon the volunteers. Both our new workers seemed committed to the work and philosophy of the Clinics and saw their remit as being to help us to maintain an efficient service and to develop our aims and objectives more fully. They both attended a training course and within a few weeks the Nursing Officer was actively participating and sharing in the workload of the Clinic sessions, policy meetings and study evenings, and the Clerical Officer was handling tasks such as organising rotas, supplies and leaflets. At Wythenshawe long awaited equipment such as labelled files, new cups and saucers and filing cabinets suddenly began miraculously to appear. Volunteers no longer found themselves having to liaise directly with the Health Authority and as consequence policy meetings became shorter and less frustrating for all concerned. Telephone calls, too, no longer presented problems because the Nursing Officer [being permanently based at the Clinic premises,] could deal with them herself.

As had been anticipated the Nursing Officer was soon to make her own assessment of how best to encourage health visitors to become involved in the Wythenshawe Clinic, and before long our training programmes were attended by several interested health visitors from other areas of Wythenshawe. Within six months of her arrival we found ourselves being joined by a group of six health visitors who took it in turns to attend the Clinic once every 4–6 weeks, and a new batch of lay volunteers.

Voluntary organisations often experience a high turnover of personnel and, by chance, the arrival of new workers coincided with impending departures of some of the most active and central figures from both Clinics. It had been observed with satisfaction that amongst both professionals and volunteers at the Clinic there had been growth of self-awareness and self-confidence. In many cases this had contributed to a need of the workers for career progression to positions allowing a further employment of their talents, more formal recognition of worth and, for the volunteers, a salary.

To make matters worse the remaining staff suffered a decline in morale which, in retrospect, stemmed from a general lack of communication. Although the arrival of more health professionals was welcomed, subsequent underlying tensions at policy meetings led to a failure to hold full and open discussion, and a sense of 'them and us' prevailed amongst the volunteers. With an increased amount of business demanding her attention the Nursing Officer experienced considerable stress, and the volunteers felt that this made it increasingly difficult for her to maintain the non-hierarchial form of the Well Woman Clinic, with decisions affecting their work being taken without their full participation. Lack of communication made it impossible to develop a teamwork approach based on mutual support and encouragement, and this precipitated a drift away from Clinic activities by both lay and professional workers, and the crisis forced us to examine why we were finding it so difficult to work together.

It emerged from the evaluation that although all parties agreed on the value of the well woman service, there was still disagreement between volunteers and health professionals concerning the degree to which the Clinic could deviate from NHS policy and practice. Again, issues such as time spent on Clinic activities and male staff and clients were raised, as was the 'political' nature of our connections with other organisations. Overall however, there was a general sense of frustration that the already considerable amount of time and effort that everybody required and expected of each other was still apparently insufficient for progress beyond simply maintaining Clinic sessions. In short, it became obvious to all concerned that there were still some serious problems that would require considerably more time and attention if the Clinics were to achieve their full potential within the Health Service. It was also obvious that no matter how sympathetic and committed the Nursing Officer was, it was impossible for her to devote the necessary time to co-ordinating and developing the service and its peculiar workforce.

In 1984 the Nursing Officer took it upon herself, therefore, to request that the Health Authority should seriously re-consider the possiblity of appointing a full-time co-ordinator. On the basis of a report that she has presented to the Authority we were informed that they were prepared to do just that, and a co-ordinator was apponted in 1985.

Overall, our experience has shown that it is possible to provide a service that responds to the self-perceived needs of its public but that attempts at integrating that service and its ideas into the Health Service as a whole, has until now produced more than a token in response to persistent pressure. Recognition of the potential of well woman clinics has, to some extent, taken place within Health Service Management, but response by the majority of health workers at other levels has placed serious doubts upon the future of such clinics unless some action is taken which recognises the underlying causes of our isolation.

Currently, the main problem is the inevitable incestuous and difficult relationship between the Clinics and the Health Service, and this is linked to the fact that they represent two different organisational structures, which, in turn stem from two different philosophies: one, hierarchial and used to definite lines of accountability, bounded by the necessity to be a political football and seen as complying with circulars and statutes, and the other, operating without a hierarchy and through participation, convinced of the political nature of health and complying with the views of women about their health needs.

Some people believe that because of these fundamental differences the Clinics may never reach their full potential if they continue to exist within the Health Service. Others however remain true to the idea that at a time of increasing consumer demand and interest in the Health Service and the continually growing number of well woman clinic campaigns, the South Manchester Clinics should not give up the ground they have already been able to make.

The enthusiasm and achievements of the health visitors, doctors, the nursing officer and others who have become involved also provides some indication that the ideas and philosophy of the Clinics are not alien to all health workers. For some the opportunity to work for and with other women in a more supportive structure than is usual in the Health Service is appealing.

The future of the Well Woman Clinics in their present form

clearly depends upon whether they can, for the time being, maintain some autonomy within the present structure of the NHS. It remains to be seen whether the appointment of a suitably qualified, full-time co-ordinator is considered to be as important to the Health Authority as it is to those of us who worked for three and a half years without one.

References

An Evaluation of the Manchester Well Woman Clinics. March 1982 (Copies of each are available from Manchester CHCs, St Ann's Churchyard, St. Ann's Street, Manchester. Tel. 061 832 8182)
Illich I (1975) *Medical Nemesis*. London: Calder & Boyers.
Newman GF (1984) *The Nations Health*. London: Granada
World Health Organisation (1978) *Alma Ata Declaration*. Geneva: WHO
Well Woman Clinic: Proposals for Manchester. June 1981. Manchester CHCs, available as above

Chapter 8

THE MANCHESTER EXPERIENCE II: WITHINGTON WELL WOMAN CLINIC

Joan Armstrong

Background

Withington Well Woman Clinic began because three colleagues shared an interest in women's health. However, in our role as family health visitors our work with women tended to be limited mainly to mothers of pre-school children. We were aware that the majority of the female population do not fit into this narrowly-defined group. We were also conscious that for the past decade women had become increasingly interested and questioning about their health and were refusing to accept that the vagaries and malfunctioning of their bodies generally, and their reproductive systems in particular, were conditions that had to be quietly tolerated as they had been for generations.

This new found assertiveness and knowledge was demonstrated in magazine and newspaper articles and in the embryonic women's health movement growing throughout the country. It seemed to us that one area where it was not evident was the place most obviously involved with the delivery of both curative and preventive medicine, namely the NHS. This anomaly seemed the more curious since the vast majority of workers of all disciplines in the NHS are women – the most notable and perhaps crucial, exception being the medical profession.

Through living and working in Withington, we already knew

a number of local women who had a commitment to, and knowledge of, women's health. They shared our conern at the lack of a comprehensive service for all women and offered to give support and practical help for any ideas we had of developing such a service.

The local Child Health Centre is in an old four-storey semi-detached house: several generations of local babies have attended the Baby Clinic. However, there were times during the week when the building was unused. The house itself has an informal atmoshpere and does not convey the image of the modern, impersonal GP-dominated health centre. The surrounding neighbourhood is a long-established residential area, originally a village and still retaining a keen sense of community. The inhabitants are socially and racially mixed: all age groups are represented as are a variety of living arrangements, from the conventional two-parent family and extended family network to people living singly, and in mixed-sex and single-sex communal houses.

The housing stock also contains a whole range of types of properties reflecting their occupants' place in the Registrar General's Classification. There is, in the lower socio-economic range unmodernised council property where many materially and socially-deprived people live, including unsupported mothers and isolated elderly women. Rising through the Classification are newly-built council properties, owner-occupied small and large terraced homes and semi-detached houses with gardens, while at the southern borders of the district may be found the large detached houses, with their own grounds, of the senior professional and managerial classes.

In another part of the Health District is a vast council estate at Wythenshawe. A Well Woman Clinic staffed by community medical officers and lay workers was opened there in 1981, the popularity of which highlighted the enormous need felt by women of all ages for the service they were being offered. We each visited the Clinic on separate occasions but came to the same conclusions afterwards that the admirable attempt to be informal had led to a lack of organisation which benefited neither clients nor workers, and that an 'open door' policy could, due to lack of space, result in some women being interviewed without privacy, and in a very long waiting time for many clients. Our visits were a useful exercise: not only did these give us ideas but the fired our enthusiasm further and confirmed our belief that this was a service which health visitors should be helping to provide in their role of health professionals in the wider community context.

Plans and concepts

The most important service we thought we could give each client was to allow her time and privacy to consider her physical health in relation to other aspects of her life and to all the other factors and people which that involved. This process was to be facilitated by an empathetic woman worker using a questionnaire as a tool. This had seemed to us to be the core philosophy behind the Wythenshawe Well Woman Clinic and one which we sought to emulate. Another important factor was demystifying medical knowledge, allowing women to become participators in the entire clinic procedure rather than behave as submissive subjects of medical experts. We had come to realise that, despite our qualifiications and experience as health visitors we did not have a deep knowledge of all aspects of women's health. For example, we had not met a sufficient number of women experiencing menopause symptoms to be able to appreciate the complexity of the situation, and our contribution to alleviate their needs was, as a result, limited. Our expensive. drug-orientated training had completely cut us off and made us suspicious of alternative forms of medicine, including treatment for many common female complaints. Some of the interested lay workers possessed this variety of knowledge and we thought their contribution to a women's health clinic was of equal value to ours. In other words, we believed that professional health workers could work alongside women in the community, sharing skills and ideas. An obvious corollary to this was the philosophy of arriving at administrative and management policy decisions in a shared, consensus manner. To those of us conditioned for many years to the hierarchical structure of the nursing profession, the concept of collective responsibility with its lack of individual leadership was a revoluntionary step which required a psychological gear change.

We put out thoughts to our line management who, in principle, agreeed. The community medical staff who are working at

Wythenshawe also supported us and were willing to work with us.

Planning the practicalities

We set about planning the practical deails of the organisation, as we considered it of prime importance in a new venture with new concepts to be prepared adequately to provide the most efficient service. The mundane, but time-consuming, tasks of deciding what equipment, stationary, and so on, were necessary, ordering them and collecting them were done. We thought that ten new clients by appointment, per afternoon session once a week, was a viable number. We allowed half to one hour for each woman to complete the questionnaire and therefore felt that three workers would be required for this role. We also thought it would be necessary to have a worker at each session whose role would be to peform clinical checks, ensure the smooth running of the session, be available to answer the queries of women 'dropping in', and reassuring the clients during the waiting phases of their visit. We were aware that any or all of these plans might need modification once the clinic was in operation.

A month before our planned opening we convened a meeting of all women who had expressed an interest in working with us. From this meeting a pool of workers from a variety of backgrounds and experience was established. A few of the volunteers had paramedical or nursing training but all shared a common interest in providing a comprehensive service to women. Posters were made and distributed locally. Our concern at this stage was – would we have any clients? Later experience proved our concern to be unfounded for once the Clinic opened in June 1982 we were overwhelmed by requests for help and information.

The Clinic session

Each woman is seen by appointment. As most appear apprehensive on arrival, and obviously taken aback by their first impression, we try to create a relaxed comfortable atmosphere. A free cup of tea made by women from a local voluntary organisation identifies the Clinic as being different from a conventional clinic waiting room. We hope that this environment encourages women to browse through the available literature and to talk to the other women in the room.

The woman is welcomed by a worker who, after initial introductions explains the clinic procedure and asks her for certain basic health information: height, weight (clients are only weighed at their own request because for women with a weight or eating problem, the act of being weighed publicly can be humiliating and embarrassing) and blood pressure; her urine is also tested.

At this point the woman is given a Health Questionnaire (see Appendix) and a Feedback Questionnaire for completion at home and return to the clinic (the constructive criticisms received via the latter have been most useful in the continuing evaluation of the clinic's work). The health questionnaire is the main document of record; it accompanies the woman during her visit and information is added to it by the workers she sees.

The next stage consists of a private interview with a worker at which they complete the health questionnare together. The questionnaire is designed to enable the woman to review her physical health from top to toe, to allow her to discuss the relationships in all areas of her life and to discuss her life style and patterns of behaviour. There is therefore no aspect of her life to which she does not have to give some attention and no aspect, however minor, is considered to be unimportant. It is this service that we claim is unique: time given by informed, empathetic women to enable oher women to identify in a calm, quiet environment the areas in their lives with which they are having difficulty, to relate this to their lives in total and to assess future action, thus enabling them to see for themselves how to acquire whole health. Women usually identify some specific issue as being their main area of concern quite early in this interview and many, by the end, will realise that some other aspect of their life may be the primary cause of their concern or distress.

It should be emphasised, however, that this questionnaire is only a tool. There are situations where its use in inappropriate, eg. when a woman on the day of attendance presents with an overwhelming single problem. It is not the same as, and requires different skills for, the history taking to which health professionals are accustomed. It is written in the woman's own words and she checks its accuracy on completion: it belongs to her and she can request its removal or destruction at any time.

Having built up this overrall picture of the whole person, the woman is asked if she would like to consult the doctor. Often, talking through her health profile satisfies the needs which initially motivated the woman to attend the Clinic. However, a large number of women do avail themselves of this opportunity to have medical queries answered in more detail and/or to have the range of checks and tests which only a doctor can undertake or authorise. Should treatment be necessary the woman is referred to her GP, who otherwise is not informed by the clinic of her attendance.

Other women may want to see a counsellor to receive guidance about emotional difficulties. This counselling is always undertaken on another occasion as it is thought to be too painful for a woman to undergo this process and the clinic visit on the same day. Two counsellors work for the Clinic: one is medically as well as marrriage-guidance trained, and to her we refer primarily woman with medically-related emotional problems, eg. eating disorders. The second counsellor is trained in general counselling skills and works on a voluntary basis: to her we refer primarily women with relationship problems.

At the end of her visit the woman is given a health record card which she retains. On it are recorded her measurements, the results of any tests she may have had and, if she has seen the doctor, recommended treatment and/or advice (all repeated from the health questionnaire). The purpose behind this is to reassure the woman that she has complete knowledge of everything that has been recorded about her during her visit. She is further assured that the whole process is confidential and that her health questionnaire when filed at the end of the session, can only be identified by number.

Organisation

The Clinic session is organised so that six new clients can be seen in an afternoon, in addition to those making return visits. Appointments are made in groups of three allowing one hour between each group, and three workers are allocated per session to interview two women each: should someone arrive requesting to be seen urgently, she will also be seen. While the first three women are with their individual worker the doctor will see those who have re-appointments, eg. women returning after a month with complete premenstrual syndrome charts or women requesting smears who are menstruating on their initial visit.

The role of the 'waiting room' worker developed as we had originally envisaged it but with the increased responsibility of ensuring, with help from the other workers, that the clinic rooms are prepared and tidied afterwards. She was also responsible for all the administrative aspects of the session. Since this role involved clinical checks, those of us who were professionals offered to teach these skills to the lay workers to ensure that everyone could share every working role. However, the lay workers collectively decided that taking blood pressure was a skill they preferred to leave to those trained and experienced in doing it, and consequence this particular task is usually peformed by a health visitor.

Due to financial constraints the Clinic session is held during working hours, and the clinic premises cannot at present be used on a regular basis in the evenings. We are, however, aware that many women take time off work to attend and there is obviously a need for an evening session.

Continuing the theme of worker role-sharing, all decisions about the clinic are taken at monthly policy meetings at which all workers are expected to attend. Ideas for development and other issues are discussed and the consensus view prevails. Requests for speakers at lay and professional meetings are dealt with. Clinic procedures are constantly reviewed, eg. the health questionnaire has been revised several times; the number of women seen and the catchment area from which we can accept them have been based on meeting decisions. No individual worker has the authority to make a decision without the meeting's approval. For the nurses among us this has proved to be an exciting, novel and refreshing form of management which, most importantly, can be seen to work.

The philosophy and practice of both Clinics has been set out in a joint policy document formulated and agreed by all the workers. This also lays down that the present general structure of the clinics cannot be altered except by resolution of an Annual General Meeting.

An early policy decision was that workers should have lunch

together before the afternoon session to increase the feeling of social cohesiveness and provide mutual support. Visitors who have shown an interest in the clinic and wish to discuss it further are also invited to this lunch. As a result, we have met people from all parts of the country, particularly members of Community Health Councils who have, we hope, benefitted from the sharing of knowledge and ideas in their attempts to start well woman clinics elsewhere.

For one reason or another many of our workers have had to move on and it is a necessary and continuing process to be seeking new recruits. We are keenly aware of the need to provide the most skilled and efficient service that is within our capabilities, and to this end we have devised a training course, which is constantly under review, of eight evenings and one day to which all new workers, whatever their background, must attend before commencing work; these sessions are guided mainly by established workers, with some assistance from outside 'experts'. We also have study and social evenings for all workers as a method of continually upgading our knowledge and getting to know each other better. All of this activity is shared with Wythenshawe Clinic workers, for from the beginning we have had a high reward for the value of close contact between the two Clinics and for the preservation of a similar philosophy and practice.

Developments and difficulties

As time has gone by, a difficulty has arisen which was not thought through at the planning stage – the constant turnover of workers. Voluntary workers take up paid employment, or other areas of their lives claim priority, and professionals, whose base enabled them originally to give a working commitment also move to new posts. Of course, alternative voluntary and professional workers offer their time and services but continual vigilance is required by the whole group to ensure that the original philosophy and practice is kept intact.

An unforeseen role we have discovered is providing an unofficial 'phone-in' service. Women from all the surrounding districts of Manchester telephone requesting appointments. As it is our policy to see only those women from our own health district we then have to listen to women, often very distressed, explaining how they feel physically and emotionally. If immediate advice can be given we do so, but our aim, apart from listening, is to refer them to another, more local, agency who we hope will be able to help with the presenting problem. This can sometimes involve trying to give a woman the confidence and reassurance to face an unsympathetic GP. All the health visitors based in the Child Health Centre, whether or not they are active in the clinic sessions, see it as their function to deal with these calls. Although we hope that these women obtain some value from the time we give them, we are nevertheless dissatisifed to have to provide such a partial service. When appropriate, we generally advise the women to contact their local Community Health Council and/or District Health Authority on the need they have experienced for a clinic in their area. Indeed, during the past 12 months more clinics have commenced in the North West.

When the Clinic had been in operation for about a year it became clear that the actual and potential volume of work was greater than the time the women involved could give to it. It was felt that to provide anything approaching an adequate service a full-time worker was required who could deal with the increasing clerical, administrative and general information demands which has so quickly arisen. It was also thought necessary to have a single 'phone'-in' point for both clinics, from where this proposed worker could give sensitive and accurate information, thus reducing the burden on the health visitors.

Conclusion

There is little doubt that this unique service provided by women for women is fulfilling a need and gaining momentum as a movement. Although practice may vary in different localities the philosophy is firmly rooted in women becoming active participants in their health care and being involved in achieving their optimum health. This will fundamentally change the concept of health care within the NHS. As for Withington Well Woman Clinic, we will continue to ask for the creation of a post for a woman to work full-time as an anchor and resource person, to ensure that the organisation and administrative aspects run smoothly and to facilitate the development of self-help groups, a central 'phone-in' service, and training sessions. Most importantly, we will be responsive to any other ideas which arise from the needs of women.

Chapter 9

THE MANCHESTER EXPERIENCE III: RUSHOLME WELL WOMAN CLINIC

Merryn Cooke . Clare Ronalds

In 1983 a well woman clinic was established as a two-year trail project within a general practice in Central Manchester. This chapter, written by two of the workers involved, describes how and why it was set up and the type of work carried out, as well as some of the difficulties encountered.

The practice area

Rusholme and Moss Side lie three miles to the south of Manchester city centre and are part of an inner city area where there is high unemployment and social deprivation. They form an area of great cultural variety and social mobility.

The main shopping street in Rusholme displays the variety; at three o'clock in the morning you will find the chippy, an Indian restaurant and the Greek kebab house all still serving customers. To one side of the main street are large Victorian houses and some 1930s semi-detached houses; many have been converted into flats although some are still occupied by families. A high proportion of Manchester's Asian population live in this area, often with three generations in one household. On the other side are the rows of pre-1919 terraced houses with cobbled paths separating the small backyard. This is a changing area with some houses being renovated, other awaiting demolition and, in between, new pockets of two-storey council housing. On the edge of Moss Side are some 1960 tower blocks. The condition of much of the housing is poor: overcrowding, damp and cockroaches are everyday problems.

The local people are mainly working class and there are sizeable ethnic minorities from Ireland, the Punjab, Bangladesh, the West Indies and Africa. Because the area is close to the University there is a large student population, many from overseas. The proportion of single-parent families is well above the city average, though the number of elderly is below average. Male unemployment is now a devastating 30% and few families own a car or telephone. The population is highly mobile. It is an area of high medical and social need.

The Robert Darbishire Practice

The practice is unusual in that the general practitioners are also lecturers in the University of Manchester Department of General Practice. The Robert Darbishire Practice, the acedemic department and the community health services are housed in a new, purpose-built health centre. A wide range of community services and clinics are available at the health centre. The Robert Darbishire Practice runs its own antenatal, immunisation and child development clinics; it has patient-participation groups, an over-60's group and a mother-and-toddler group, which all meet weekly. It employs a practice nurse and has attached health visitors and a psychiatric social worker.

There is one full-time, general practitioner and the other seven doctors work in three teams. Only one of the principals is a woman and thus only the patients of one team have potential access to a woman GP. Four trainees, some of whom are female are attached to the practice, one to each team, for a year at a time.

The practice population of approximately 12,000 patients has two unusual features: a very high turnover (about 20% of the patients change each year) and a high proportion of 18-to-25-year olds.

Background to the Clinic

Many of the problems that the local people have to live with are a complex interaction, not only of health and illness, but of social, economic and cultural factors. The two health visitors and the woman GP were convinced that women could be helped by more health information and discussion than is possible in conventional surgery consultations, and that they might benefit from an opportunity to explore problems such as tiredness in a different setting which would enable them to look for alternative solutions to the medical ones. A resource centre and meeting place were needed where women could meet in a comfortable environment, obtain health advice and information and talk to other women about their problems.

From 1981, when the first woman doctor was appointed to the practice, a proportion of women patients had the choice of consulting a woman doctor and, later, more women patients sought that same access. There was concern, particularly by the health visitors, that the lack of availability of a woman doctor might prevent some women from seeking advice, especially for embarrassing problems such as cervical smears and breast disorders. Furthermore, we were aware that our local population is predominantly from social classes, IIIM, IV and V, and use the preventive health services least and yet have greater health risks than those in higher social classes.

For all these reasons we decided to set up a women's clinic whose aims were:

(i) to give women an opportunity to talk to other women about problems;
(ii) to give women patients an option to see a woman doctor;
(iii) to help women learn about their bodies and how to keep healthy;
(iv) to offer health information and advice, including alternatives to conventional medicine;
(v) to offer preventative health services, eg. cervical smears.

Setting up the Clinic

We thought that ideally such a clinic should be provided for all women in the area and be based in a familiar environment. Two well woman clinics already existed in South Manchester and a campaign for a clinic had been started in Central Manchester. Listening to local women at campaign meetings confirmed our impression that there were needs unmet by the existing Health

Service. Approaches were made by the health visitors and woman general practitioner to the Central District Community Health Authorities about starting a well woman clinic. It became clear that there was no support for such a clinic being established in Central Manchester. The District Management Team felt that the services currently available to women were adequate, and did not wish to offend local general practitioners, believing that there was a conflict between the well woman clinic and the traditional general practioner's role. Far from believing this, we thought that a clinic would complement the work of general practitioners.

The practice-based workers decided that one option was to organise a clinic as part of their general practice work. Since it was to be in this setting it could only be available to women registered with the Robert Darbishire Practice, it would not be publically advertised and had to be held on practice premises. The nursing management agreed to the health visitors being involved in a well woman clinic in this setting and the practice partners consented to the service being offered to their patients for a trail period of one year.

The health visitors contacted other possible workers, eg. the district midwife, the practice social worker, and other colleagues who were known to have an interest in women's health. The response from the volunteers was amazing and a list of those willing to help run the clinic included nurses and nurse lecturers, health visitors, a midwife, a psychiatric social worker, a psychologist, a counsellor, community workers from the Asian Women's Refuge who offered to provide translators, and a woman general practitioner from outside Manchester who had written and researched extensively on the menopause.

We then collected health education material from variety of sources. After two planning meetings and with minimal publicity we opened the clinic. In our efforts to present a relaxed atmosphere we had no formal clinic procedure. We decided not to use an interview schedule or questionnaire because black women, in particular, strongly objected to these.

Developments

The eighteen months since the clinic opened were a period

of continuous assessment and change. Problems arose almost immediately. Some people were unsure of their role in the clinic, of how much medical knowledge they should have, of their own counselling skills and of the role of the doctors in the well woman setting. The difficulties arose partly because the volunteers were co-opted after the initial planning of the clinic, and partly because there was a lack of training or discussion meetings at the start. However, the informal clinic structure and lack of hierarchy, as well as the closeness of the majority of the workers who saw each other daily in the health centre, made it easy for them to share their problems.

Consequently, monthly lunchtime and evening meetings were arranged where general policy, as well as specific topics, were discussed. The meetings were too infrequent and volunteers from otuside the practice still felt isolated. In our second year we met weekly on the morning after the clinic: this improved communication, but there were still problems in integrating outside volunteers with those from the practice.

Most workers have had some formal training in the health field but in many ways this training does not help us to make patients more autonomous, to impart knowledge or skill to others or to help patients to explore senstive or embarrassing issues. Although one woman went to the ten-week training session run by the South Manchester Well Woman Group, the only training most volunteers had was six one-hour sessions as well as using some of the weekly meetings to discuss issues arising from work in the clinic – topics such as breast cancer, depression, or alternative therapies. The provision of more training did not prove feasible due to lack of volunteers' time, and because our weekly meetings were more concerned with policy than with educational issues.

Initially, most workers felt unsure of their role when interviewing women. Should they only discuss what the woman brought up or should they initiate discussion on a more general basis and if so, how and on what? Although we did not want a long, formal questionnaire we decided to have a short open-ended checklist which was to be an aide-memoire for the volunteers. On this we recorded the woman's name, address, age and general practitioner and a short summary checklist which includes questions on the menstrual cycle, diet, sexual relationships, emotional state and sleeping patterns. Anything written down was agreed with the woman herself. The doctor's notes were also recorded on the checklist. Information about physical examinations, tests ordered or prescriptions given was transferred to the woman's medical records which were available for the doctors.

A major problem we encountered is one which is still being debated within the many and varied well woman groups in the country – that of sharing power and expertise between patient, volunteer and doctor. One of our aims was to demedicalise many aspects of women's health problems, to give women time to explore the links between social and emotional pressures and ill health, and to give them the confidence and skills to take responsibility for their health and get the best from the NHS.

Many women came to the clinic to see the woman doctor for a specific medical problem, and did not wish to explore more personal issues. However, when a doctor is available volunteers are always tempted to refer or suggest to women that they could see her, especially where, as in our clinic, the woman doctor is an able and willing counsellor. Many women attending the clinic come with a medical problem as a 'ticket' to legitimise their visit when their real reason may be social or psychological. The volunteer who is unsure of her level of knowledge may collude with a woman who is unsure whether to explore painful or worrying feelings, and both may agree that the doctor can solve the problem.

Whilst the doctor is there to provide technical resources, such as assessing the appropriateness of hormone replacement therapy for menopausal symptoms, our belief is that much of the counselling work is best done by people other than the doctors. By sharing experiences with other women who have some understanding and awareness of the problems but who are not medically qualified we hope patients can be enabled to help themselves. Learning to judge when it is appropriate to refer to the doctor has been difficult. The tendency has been for the volunteers to be over-cautious and under-estimate their own abilities. We wanted the health education and self-help role of the Clinic to be developed more than the medical and screening role but it has been difficult to achieve this: obeisance to the medical hierarchy is still powerful for patients, doctors and volunteers. All the clinic workers have been conscious of this problem and struggled to counteract it and retain a democratic structure.

The female practice population is approximately 5,000 (aged 16 upwards). On average four women were seen per clinic session and the low numbers caused concern among the workers, especially on evenings when no-one turned up. For medicolegal reasons we could not advertise the clinic outside the practice so we informed registered patients of our existence by postal leaflets, practice posters and information to potential referers. The drawbacks to this were that the posters only reached women who entered the health centre for postage was limited. Thus, using the age/sex register, we sent duplicated leaflets in English and three Asian languages to the 40–50 age group of women patients and laboriously addressed envelopes. Later, we mailed all 35–40-year-old women, using the practice computer to select patients and print labels. The posters for the reception area stressed that ample time would be available to talk to other women in confidence and that health information and screening facilities are provided. Perhaps the most successful method of informing potential clients was to ask doctors, receptionists, community nursing staff and other workers to mention our existence to women who might be interested. Some doctors have asked the women's clinic to counsel particular patients who they felt needed more time than could be given in a normal consultation, and also offered women the choice of seeing the woman doctor for cervical smears.

As the clinic is restricted to patients registered with the practice we were unsure of what to do should women from outside it come for help. In fact, this has only happened a few times and women who enquired were advised about possible sources of help and given the address of the nearest district well woman clinic. In two cases the women were extremely distressed and did need urgent attention – they were seen by the doctor and referred immediately to their own GP.

We have tried to expand the educational role of the Clinic by collecting leaflets and articles, eg. about premenstrual tension and the menopause. We have made two videotapes, one on breast self-examination and the other about hysterectomy, and have borowed some from the Health Education Council. The practice gave us £50 to buy reference books, which have been well used by patients and workers.

Although many of the videotapes available from the Health Education Council were very interesting and informative it required time and commitment to sort through catalogues, book the tapes, advertise when they would be shown collect and take them back and set up equipment. It was therefore frustrating if no-one turned up at the clinic, and there was no guarantee that those who did come would wish to see the videotape being shown. We realised that it would be better to put the effort into making our own or wait until there were more women interested in a particular subject.

How the Clinic works

The Clinic is open from 5pm to 7pm every Monday evening. We have the use of five rooms; a large room with chairs and tables where we have the video and leaflets, a playroom next door with toys, a doctor's consulting room and two small interview rooms. There are usually four volunteers on duty at each session, including either a woman doctor or a midwife who could take a cervical smear should a patient request one. There is now a doctor present for three out of every four sessions. Once a month another female doctor with a special interest in the menopause and women's health works at the clinic. We have an examination trolley for the doctor's room and another one which contains health information.

Women arriving at the clinic for the first time often have only a vague idea of its function. We therefore try to make the atmosphere as friendly and relaxed as possible, give a clear explanation of what we offer and give the woman a chance to ask questions.

One worker welcomes the woman, offers tea of coffee and talks to her at one end of the reception room. If she has childen another worker will play with them in the crêche next door. The following is the check-list that volunteers then go through:

1 Check that the woman is registered at the practice.
2 Explain what we offer:
   Time to talk
   Help in looking at general health via the interview schedule
   The opportunity to see a woman doctor,
   Screening tests such as blood pressure, urine, weight, breast examination and cervical smear
   Leaflets, books and videos

3 Explain who the workers are.
4 Explain that the conversations are confidential except for what is written in medical records.
5 Give the woman a chance to ask questions.

We offer all women the opportunity to talk privately to one volunteer, even if it is only to clarify what she wants to say to a doctor. If a woman has a specific problem we try to arrange for her to talk to a volunteer with that particular interest and expertise. During the interview the volunteer may go through the check list with the woman or simply discuss a particular problem; she will offer routine screening tests. If the woman decides to see the doctor the volunteer will go with her if she wishes. Follow-up is arranged on an individual basis.

The women seen at the Clinic

About 70 new patients were seen during the first year within a total of about 140 visits: on average, we saw four women each session. Although the age range was wide, the majority of the women were between 20 and 35. They presented with a great variety of problems: as expected, we saw women with cystitis, hot flushes, or premenstrual tension, and also those requesting information on many topics including contraception, especially after publicity on the links between cancer and the Pill. A number of women came for screening, eg. cervical smears or blood-pressure checks. In most cases there were long-standing underlying problems that they wished to discuss. Sexual problems were common and it was important that volunteers should be aware of the likelihood of these difficulties and feel comfortable enough to raise the subject and discuss it with them.

It was also clear that some women with long-standing problems which had not improved with conventional treatment were looking to the clinic for reassurance that they were not 'over-reacting, neurotic or demanding'. These women often wanted information on the effectiveness and availability of alternative therapies that they had read about or seen on television. Some of the male doctors in the practice offered their female patients the opportunity to see the woman doctor if they needed an internal examination. Some patients with embarrassing symptoms came to us before consulting their own GP. We provided a useful service for those who for cultural reasons, eg. Muslim women who wish to see a female doctor.

The following case histories illustrate some of the problems presented and how they were dealt with.

Holly

Holly came to the clinic in April. She was hoping to marry soon and wished to discuss contraception. She spoke to one of the workers for half an hour and together they produced a list of her problems, which included anxieties about her wedding night, sexual intercourse, contraception and lower abdominal pain. She asked if she could have cervical smear as she had never had one. It became clear that she was unfamiliar with her own body and that this was leading to anxiety about sex and penetration. Before going in with her to see the doctor the volunteer showed Holly a speculum and a diagram of the uterus and vagina and explained what would happen if she had an internal examination and a smear was taken. Following the initial interview Holly, the volunteer and the doctor spent an hour discussing the issues, including contraception options. She was also taught breast self-examination. She was given a pelvic examination which reassured her that all was normal and by using a mirror she was able to see herself, which helped to reduce some of her ignorance and fear of intercourse.

Mary

Mary heard about the clinic from her general practitioner and came requesting a routine cervical smear. She had seen her own doctor two weeks previously about contraception and had changed to a low-progesterone pill because she was worried about the media reports on the association between oral contraception and cancer. She was seen in the clinic by a worker who went through the interview schedule with her. She had recently changed her job to be a secretary in a publishing firm, work which she found stressful.

She was attempting to give up smoking and was encouraged, by sharing anti-smoking ideas, to continue doing this although it was a difficult time of her life. She was asked about her diet and replied that she felt overweight. She was weighed, and at 14 stone (88.9 kg) was 2.5 stone (15.88 kg) above her ideal weight. She and the counsellor talked about diet and exercise. Interestingly, when she was then seen by the woman doctor she did not ask for a routine smear but said she had noticed lumps in her vagina which worried her: examination showed that she had vaginal warts and a discharge. A routine cervical smear, the original entrance ticket to the clinic, was also carried out. She was taught breast self-examination as part of that check up. It was seen from her medical notes that she had raised blood pressure: this was checked in the clinic and found to be lower. She was referred to the sexually-transmitted diseases clinic for treatment for her multiple warts. This 'I've just come for a smear' presentation in fact resulted in Mary being given support and health information as well as a diagnosis for an embarrassing medical condition.

Edith

Edith was in her early 50s and wanted to know whether she was menopausal. She complained that she was tired, irritable and could not get on with people at work or at home. She wished to see the doctor and did not want an initial interview. In a long consultation with the doctor it transpired that she had major psychosexual problems. She also suffered from stress incontinence and wondered whether all her symptoms were attributable to the menopause. Furthermore, she wanted to share the difficulty she had in explaining menstruation and sex to her daughter as she felt unable to discuss this with her friends. Examination showed that she had a cystocele and she was referred to her own GP for a gynaecological referral. After a long discussion she was offered an opportunity for further psychosexual counselling with the psychiatric social worker or the Marriage Guidance Service. She was given leaflets about the menopause and an open invitation to return to see the videotape. She had in the past been labelled as anxious and insecure and 'requiring advice as to whether she was bringing up the family well or not'. Her desire for more information and need to share her feelings about what to tell her daughter did not seem inappropriate to us.

Two Ladies

We saw fewer patients with menopause problems than we expected. One evening two ladies came, one as a support for her friend, to talk about the 'change of life' and its devastating effect on their lives. They spent a long time talking to one of the volunteers who had carried out research into the effects of the menopause. Following this general discussion they looked at our videotape on hysterectomy and subsequent early menopause. The film mentioned sexual problems and this prompted the two women to talk about this aspect of their lives too. They returned for a further discussion with two of the workers the following week. The group discussion seemed to be an interesting development and one which we would like to pursue. Certainly at women's health courses held locally, discussion groups on the menopause are always well attended but there may not be enough women within our practice who would want to attend one at the clinic.

Long-term Counselling

A number of women have come, or been referred by their doctors, for longer-term counselling on physical symptoms such as insomnia, backache or rashes which relate to an underlying depression or anxiety. These women have usually attended for a few weeks and then once every few months for some supportive help in crises.

Christine, a divorcee with a stressful job and financial problems which made her feel guilty that she could not give her teenage children the kind of material things she wanted them to have, had a very difficult relationship with a new partner. In the first four sessions whe was able mainly to express her various distresses and ventilate her problems about the situation. She was then seen twice in the next six months on occasions when she had a crisis with her boyfriend. At the end of this time it became clear that the situation was deteriorating and she decided that she needed to explore her own behaviour further and was thus referred from the clinic for psychotherapy.

Surinder had two young children and her husband was unemployed and drank. He had been violent to her and during the session she was able to say that he often forced her to have intercourse against her will. She felt isolated and quite unable to talk about sexual matters with anyone in her community but at the clinic could relax and express her unhappiness and talk of the options available to her. She has stayed with her husband but now has the support of the health visitor and the Well Woman Clinic should she need it, and also knows of the existence of the Asian Women's Refuge.

Pauline had a vaginal discharge and consulted her GP about it; after several visits to him she revealed that she had been sexually abused as a child. He referred her to the Well Woman Clinic. She had never talked of the abuse and the counsellor encouraged her to describe what had happened, to talk about her present problems with her family and husband and to explore whether or not to tell them about her experience. She was also lent books and articles written by women who had also been sexually abused which, she said, made her feel much less isolated, guilty and ashamed and helped to validate her feelings of anger. She was also given the telephone number of a local group of Incest Survivors which had just started in Manchester, should she wish to talk further.

Jane suffered from long-term depression and anxiety and had a history of back pain and premenstrual tension. She hated taking drugs. Apart from exploring her social situation she was given advice on diet, alternative remedies and the address of the homeopathic clinic, where she then registered. She decided to learn yoga and meditation.

Mrs R. Mrs R. has several children and an alcoholic husband and came to the clinic intermittently for support in times of need. She suffered from premenstrual tension, had persistent financial problems, was often tired and felt trapped in her social situation. She came when she wanted to talk about a problem, leaving her children in the playroom for an hour, had a cup of tea and talked to another adult about herself.

Occasionally, she was given practical help with her bedwetting children and a neck and shoulder massage. A few years previously Mrs R. had attended a psychiatric day centre and coming to the Clinic may help her to avoid a further depressive illness. The clinic offered her a drop-in centre, which is one of its important functions – it is a resource for women to turn to when health, financial or family problems are getting them down.

Conclusions

During the first eighteen months we came to realise the advantage and limitations of a well woman clinic in a general practice setting. Such a clinic is different from that organised by Community Medical Services for a district or from a self-help group by non-medical women. Well woman clinics vary from practice to practice: Some are cervical screening clinics, others offer combined gynaecological and family planning sessions. We wanted ours to develop a different role to promote health education, provide information and to offer opportunities for exploring health problems in relation to life events. We already have a practice providing good clinical care.

The first advantage of the clinic is that it gives every woman in the practice an option to see a woman doctor for certain (often, to them embarrassing) conditions. In this multicultural area this is particularly valuable, although there is good evidence that, in general, some women prefer to talk to a woman doctor about certain problems.

Secondly, because there are no appointments, because there is a crèche, and because the atmosphere is relaxed, women are better able to take advantage of the longer time available to talk about more sensitive problems. This has helped the practice staff, who sometimes saw that women patients had problems but were unable to help them because of the limitations of the conventional practice setting.

Thirdly, in the whole of society the distribution of power within relationships is weighted towards men and against women. This inevitably and unconsciously affects all situations, including the medical consultation. Women patients are usually the passive recipients of male-diminated health care. Thus, another advantage of a well woman clinic is that it offers and encourages a more equal relationship between women patients and the health workers. Talking comfortably to other women may give them more insight into their own situation and enable them to believe in their own ability to change things. The imbalance of power is most marked between doctors and patients. Women doctors, by their training, retain a lot of power within a doctor-patient relationship, but many women patients seek the empathy they need from women doctors.

Fourthly, the books, videotapes and leaflets are resources for local women, many of whom could not afford them nor know where to find them at the particular time they need them.

Fifthly, the accessibility of the medical records for the doctors is an undoubted asset. The ability to prescribe and to arrange tests immediately is of great advantage to the patients. However, all workers need to be sensitive to the issues of confidentiality and towards promoting the relationship between the patient and her own GP: our aim is not to undermine this work but to augment it and to enable patients to use the Health Service more effectively.

By limiting the service to registered practice patients the overall number of women attending the clinic is small. Although individual women are given a lot of help, the fact that small numbers attend each week is frustrating for volunteers, who feel underused. There is less incentive to develop new ideas and resources and it is painful to have to turn away women in obvious need who are not registered.

The second major disadvantage is that it is extremely difficult to de-medicalise people's problems in a health centre setting. Although it is the philosophy of the health centre to promote health and well-being, a service is provided rather than people determining their own needs. Ideally, one should have such a resource centre organised by women themselves outside the health centre.

We hoped, by setting up a well woman clinic within a restricted practice setting, to demonstrate the need of some women in Central Manchester for such a service, and provide evidence for the local campaign for a Well Woman Clinic. We have shown that, from a practice with many facilities and with a population of about 5,000 women over 16 years of age, about four women a week are asking for help from the clinic. We could thus extrapolate from about 50,000 women in Central

Manchester, many of whom have no access of facilities in their practice, that a well woman clinic would satisfy a real need.

In the Central District of Manchester only eight of 71 general practitioners are women: Thus the majority of women cannot easily consult a female doctor. If there were more women general practitioners part of the work of a well woman clinic in a general practice setting would be superflous and the main thrust of the work could be carried out in a community centre by the women themselves, using health workers and other volunteers as resources when and how they saw fit.

Postscript

The Well Women Clinic at Rusholme Health Centre for the patients of the Robert Darbishire Practice closed in December 1984 after completing a two-year trial. Staff changes made it difficult to continue the clinic, and at review it was agreed that the attendance did not justify the current input of time and energy when priorities for the practice patients as a whole, as well as for the workers, were considered. The initiating and running of the Clinic, which was a controversial project, took a great deal of commitment from all the workers, who deserved acknowledgement and thanks for all their hard work and enthusiasm.

This report of the clinic has been compiled by the woman GP and one counsellor on behalf of the clinic workers, and we hope it reflects a consensus view of our aims, although each individual worker has a different perspective on the role of such a clinic in women's health care, and of its problems.

Finally, although the Clinic no longer exists it has, we believe, increased the awareness of the practice staff to the problems and health issues that affect women patients. It is this raised consciousness which may promote better health care and help future development.

Chapter 10

THE LIVERPOOL EXPERIENCE: THE CROXTETH WOMEN'S HEALTH GROUP: Self-help in a Deprived Community in Liverpool

Effie Sherlock

Local Initiatives in Vauxhall, Liverpool

Pat Thornley

THE CROXTETH WOMEN'S HEALTH GROUP

Croxteth is a fairly typical overspill estate built during the great slum clearance programmes of the 1950s and 60s. Over the years it has suffered the effects of poor housing maintenance, failure to develop community facilities and, more recently, soaring levels of unemployment. It has a high proportion of low-rise, deck-access-type flats and multistorey blocks. A recent report by the City's housing department identified part of the estate as being the worst in Liverpool. This area is now undergoing major refurbishment. On the rest of the estate the housing conditions continue to deteriorate, presenting a variety of public health problems: prolific damp and mould, blocked drains and sporadic outbreaks of rat infestation in or around the flats.

A report published in 1982 for the City Council highlighted the health and social problems in Croxteth. Its findings included a rising trend in the infant mortality rate and a higher than city average of low birth weight babies. The male unemployment rate was nearly 50% and the uptake of welfare benefits 81%. The report also looked at service provision. It found shortfalls in maternity services, care of the elderly, and health care for women. It was against this background that the Women's Health Group was founded. I had been gathering information and researching aspects of health and health services for the report and was asked to chair the health committee of the working party because of my health visiting background and knowledge of the area. I set out to make contact with as many of the community groups as possible, as well as talking to health and allied professionals in Croxteth. I attended numerous community groups meetings including the Tenants' Association (which met in the health clinic); the Federation of Community Groups, pensioners, and a handicap support group. It was talking to women in these groups which precipitated the formation of the Women's Health Group.

The Foundation of the Women's Health Group

A number of women from the community groups shared our concern about the state of health on the estate and a group was formed to discuss health matters. The first meeting was held at the Croxteth clinic. It had been advertised by posters and announcements at various community group meetings and 15 women attended, including myself and a community education worker – their ages ranged from the early 20s to over 60. Two main themes emerged from the discussion: the need to discuss health service provision for people in Croxteth, and an interest in discussing aspects of women's health and a sharing of experiences.

D, N and B are some of the women who attended the first meeting who are still members of the group: all live and work in Croxteth.

The Women

D is 39 years old and married, with seven children whose ages range from 10 to 21 years. D also had a handicapped child who died five years ago. She and her family have lived in Croxteth for fifteen years, currently in a four-bedroomed council house. D works at present as assistant administrator in the Croxteth Community School. She first became involved in community groups eight years ago, as a founder member of the handicap support group. It was two years ago, however, when the local comprehensive school was closed that she developed a wider interest in the community. She joined the parents' action committee, which campaigned successfully to have the school re-opened. For a time D taught in the school and did some of the administrative work. Since then she has worked in the tenants' groups, the slimmers, the Women's Health Group. She is currently in the women's jogging group, and attends weekly aerobics classes.

I spoke to the women about their views on Croxteth, themselves, and their health; this is what D had to say: '. . . I think it is living in Croxteth which gives you a vested interest in the area. Really, you want to build a better environment for the kids. Being involved in the way I am has given me a wider outlook on life. Before it was all home and the kids. Now I reckon I could give a point of view on a variety of subjects. I tend to want things to happen now. I'm never satisfied with accepting the way things are like I used to. I enjoy meeting people'.

'In the Women's Health Group I found out more about what services are available for women, for example, the well woman clinics. I've found it helpful talking about health problems that worry me and finding that other women share my concerns. I'm rarely bored these days. I feel fitter and I think I'm more confident than I used to be. I could never go back to being an ordinary housewife again . . .'

N is 28, married with four children. When the family moved to Croxteth ten years ago they lived in a second-floor flat in a walk-up block. They moved three years ago to their three-bedroomed council house. N does voluntary work at a local advice centre. She is at present on a Welfare Rights course and a Women's Health training course.

'. . . I didn't realise how isolating it is bringing up young children in a flat. I kept going to the doctor and being prescribed Valium for depression. But really it was the housing that was making me depressed. As soon as I moved to the house I felt completely different. I don't think the doctors listen to you properly. It was the same when I was pregnant. I wanted to have the baby myself, without the drip. But somehow or other once you get into the hospital it just happens and nobody explains what's happening or why. I wish I'd known then what I know now. I've learnt a lot from the discussions we've had about health. What I've found it that there are other ways of dealing with things like premenstrual tension than pills. You find out that there's a lot you can do yourself and really we know more about our own bodies than doctors. I'd like to find out more about homeopathy and alternative medicine. I think its all wrong the way doctors give out drugs like sweets . . .'

B is 45, married, with four children aged 20 to 28 years, and has lived in Croxteth for the last 32 years. She is secretary to the Federation and is probably the most knowledgeable person on community affairs in Croxteth. One of her majority contributions has been pioneering housing needs as a major community issue. Her knowledge and expertise in this field was invaluable.
'. . . I think the worst health hazards in Croxteth are bad housing, unemployment and poverty. Now, of course, there's the drug problem, too. some of the solutions can only be political. We need a strong government commitment to massive public spending on the Health Service and Council housing. I think in the Women's Health Group there has been a mutual heightening of awareness of the need for better health care and also we've learnt from each other. Because of the informality of the meetings, everybody gets a chance to speak. I think that's very important. How it will develop? I don't know. I suppose it will depend on the women who come and what they want to get out of it . . .'

Publicity – the summer carnival

At about the time of our first meeting, the community was preparing for its annual summer carnival which was to he held in July. It was felt that we should print leaflets for distribution at the carnival. We had also decided to advertise the Group by initiating a series of discussions on women's health topics, planned as a six-week women's health course, to commence in September. We agreed to continue meeting monthly in the meantime. During the summer we found that attendance varied; this, it was felt, was partly due to the summer holidays, so it was agreed that we should meet in the evenings instead. We also changed our venue to the Information Centre.

The community health workers

We received information that funds were available for a community health project and decided to apply for two community health workers. Because there was evidence that drug (heroin) abuse on the estate was reaching alarming proportions, particularly amongst teenagers, we felt that community health workers could co-ordinate and develop services locally to deal with the problem. Their remit would also be to investigate and report on health needs and the provision of services, and to produce a report for the Health Authority and the community. We put in a proposal along these lines. The workers would be managed by the Federation of Community Groups in conjunction with the Women's Health Group.

The women's health course

By now we were approaching the end of the summer. We had devised a health course drawing on topics which had been of recurrent interest in the group and I was asked to arrange for some guest speakers. We were also going to use some of the Well Woman videotape from a Channel 4 TV series.

The course began as planned at the beginning of September. It was held in the afternoon at the Clinic. Crêche facilities were available locally. The topics covered were premenstrual tension, depression, the menopause, patients' rights, hysterectomy and mastectomy. For the latter we invited members of local self-help groups to give information about support and after-care. Attendance varied from six to twenty women. On average, the women were aged between late 20s to 50s. There was a particularly good response to the discussions on premenstrual tension, menopause and depression. We began each session with either a short introduction from a guest speaker or one of the videos: this was used to trigger discussion; handouts were provided.

Campaigning for better services

During the session on patients' rights the discussion focused on the services in Croxteth. Concern was expressed about local maternity services, and the lack of a cervical cytology clinic. Both these issues were raised when the group met again. In the following weeks the discussion broadened to include other aspects of service provision. B highlighted the problems of lack of co-ordination and local provision of primary health care which had become apparent to her when her grandmother had been recently discharged from hospital into the community. Drawing the threads together from the previous discussions, the women concluded that there were a number of key areas which needed to be pursued. These were the provision of health centre facilities with particular emphasis on the need for a well-woman clinic and an antenatal clinic on the estate.

Letters with petitions were sent to the District Health Authority. We were also aware of the need for an effective national recall system for cervical cancer screening. Screening for breast cancer was also inadequately resourced. The breast screening unit at the University was able to offer a service only to women over 50 because of limited funding.

A further letter was sent to the District Health Authority highlighting the problem of the breast-screening unit. N suggested a meeting with our MP: This was arranged and subsequently a question was asked in the House about the availability of cancer screening resources for women nationally.

In the last twelve months we have seen some results from the campaign. The District Health Authority has promised a well woman clinic to commence in September. Plans to extend and improve the clinic building are scheduled to begin next year. The application for community health workers was unsuccessful, however, and there has as yet been no improvement in the provision of maternity services.

Role play

During the months of compaigning, discussion within the group continued: aspects of women's health, treatment by family doctors, and alternative approaches to health care were the main topics. Problems with doctors were a recurrent theme and many women expressed dissatisfaction after consultations because they felt they had not been listened to. There was also widespread concern about the extent to which tranquilisers were prescribed. Discussion also focused on patients' rights, health choices and the difficulties in communication between lay people and professional health workers.

At this stage we used role play to act out various situations that the women had experienced within the health service: these included exploring ways of gaining access to the GP via the receptionist, and being faced with students during examinations in hospital. In these situations feelings of helplessness and the inability to express what they wanted were described by the women. We used the role play to find different ways of reacting to the same situation. This was a particularly useful exercise; by swopping roles it also gave women an opportunity to gain an insight into the position of the health workers. The key to the exercise seemed to be the discovery of ways to be more assertive and in the future an assertiveness training course (with particular emphasis on patients' rights) may be useful.

The Sports Centre exercises and relaxation

Our meetings are held now in the newly-opened Sports Centre. The building has a well-equipped community room with a video installed. We changed venue because we included exercise and relaxation sessions, which began following the discussions on premenstrual tension. Such was the response to the relaxation exercises that we have followed this up with monthly visits to the turkish baths.

The health week

During recent months we have been busy organising a health week in Croxteth. We had provided a stall at the Summer

Carnival last year and B suggested that we should extend this to a health fair day. Ideas for a health week have developed over the last year. One of the aims of the health week is to present more opportunities for women to take part in sport and physical training activities. A community sports project and the local community programme are helping in organisation and provision of events.

It is also hoped that we will attract older people, particularly pensioners, to join in the activities, such as swimming sessions for pensioners, bowls, a keep-fit session, and a tea-dance. There will also be women's fitness training, women's self-defence, netball, tai-chi, yoga and a Look-After-Yourself course.

The Regional Health Promotion Team will be providing a health bus for the week, with fitness testing and information about lifestyle, diet and health. At the end of the week we will hold a health fair day and have planned a week to coincide with the District Health Authority's Health Carnival.

The week's activities will be followed with classes that people were particularly interested in, such as a Look-After-Yourself course; and an information catalogue of local facilities, classes and self-help groups. Publicity during the week will be enhanced by the presence of the TV Team from Brookside. There will be the winner of the Fittest Family Competition and the week will be rounded off by a 'fun-run' round a Croxteth country park.

Involvement with the Women's Health Group has been an enjoyable and enlightening experience. The warmth and humour which emerged as the women shared their experiences and knowledge enriched and broadened my own perspective of health and community life. In this type of forum participation and co-operation in learning ensues the transmission of knowledge becomes a two-way process, rather than a more didactic model of learning. This experience has illustrated the importance of approaching health promotion from the community level.

Community resource

As a health professional in this situation, there are skills and knowledge which I can contribute. My contribution is a resource to be used in response to the needs expressed by the community. There is a vast difference between this approach and the 'health expert' giving advice and teaching. Health visitors, in particular, are often in a position to act as a catalyst in a community. By the nature of our work with individual families we witness the effect of social and environmental factors on people's health. The likelihood of bringing about changes and improvements in public health is far greater with a strong community response.

Power of groups

There are other advantages, too. Bringing people together reduces the isolation that is often imposed by the type of housing that they live in. Being able to recognise common problems, and bring about change either in their own lives or those of others in the community gives them a sense of power.

The future

As far as the Group's future is concerned, there is a difficulty in maintaining a sense of continuity, mainly because of the changing composition of the Group. On reflection, this may be resolved by having a closed membership, with open meetings for special events such as the health course.

The strength of the Group has been its informal structure, size and continuing focus on health issues. One aim would be to see more women becoming involved who are not already active in other community groups, but how the Group develops depends on the current needs and concerns prevalent in the community. One possibility is to extend knowledge and skills by providing a health resource and information service, similar to a Welfare Rights service. B has attended a ten-week course on women's health training which explores this kind of venture and it is to be hoped that there may be more of these courses provided.

In any event, the group will probably continue in more or less its present form, providing a welcome opportunity for women to share their wealth of experiences and knowledge.

Reference

Croxteth Area Working Party Report. *To Look at the Needs of the Area.* 1983) Liverpool City Council.

LOCAL INITIATIVES IN VAUXHALL, LIVERPOOL

In 1982, the Vauxhall Neighbourhood Council, based in the local community centre, initiated an imaginative health promotion project. In their concern about local people's health, they sponsored one of Liverpool's first lay health workers, funded by the Manpower Services Commission. The aim was to encourage the local community, and in particular women, to develop a positive attitude to health and health care. This would enable them to develop the self-confidence necessary to make better use of the services available, and to make their unmet needs known to the health professionals.

As part of that health promotion projection, the lay health worker organised and set up locally-based women and child health courses. These covered a wide variety of topics, the emphasis being on the provision of information, advice, preventive health care, group discussion, etc. The lay worker encouraged the development of an anorexia self-help group and became actively involved in Alcoholics Anonymous and drug abuse self-help groups. She offered help and support to a group of women who, being concerned about pregnancy and childbirth, wished to set up an information support service.

A maternity information and support centre was established in June 1984, in the Vauxhall Community Centre. This offered an informal once-weekly telephone or drop-in service. The aim was to offer women information and non-medical advice on various aspects of pregnancy: home confinement, the Domino scheme and the birthing chair. As this service has professional back-up, women can be put in touch with other agencies when further information and advice is required.

The objective of the service was to help women to become more knowledgeable about their bodies and the reproductive process. Support and encouragement was given which enabled women to have the self-confidence necessary to make their needs known to the health professionals. The service was extended by making contact with local women's groups within the community and sending someone along to talk to them about it and information available, and so on.

The Vauxhall health promotion project was further extended with the employment of two additional part-time lay health workers, funded by the Manpower Services Commission; their role was to help to develop the promotion of health education and preventive health care. This was achieved by talking to women's groups, leafleting, putting together a health questionnaire for future circulation, and so on. They were also responsible for the establishment and management of a crêche facility for one-and-a-half hours each morning in the local health centre.

Since January 1985, I have also been employed as a lay health worker, sponsored by the Vauxhall Neighbourhood Council and funded by Merseyside County Council. My role is concerned with women's health, particularly that of women in the North end of Liverpool, who, for a variety of reasons, do not 'take up' the services available. A different approach to the promotion of health education and preventive health care is being developed. Although it is still orientated toward the local community, a long-term strategy is being developed and put into practice which will have spin-offs to women both locally and in the wider community. It involves the setting up of a Women's Health Information and Support Centre, the establishment of a continuing women's health training course incorporating planned updating and an eventual pilot scheme for a girls' health club.

These ideas have a threefold purpose in that it is intended (a) to develop and build on the collective skills of women in the community, (b) facilitate more effective channels of communication with sympathetic and committed professionals, and (c) develop an awareness amongst young girls in order that they may effectively influence their health in the widest sense of the word. It was felt that there were many women, both individuals and groups, who were interested or actively involved in women's health issues. There was a need to co-ordinate their ideas, activities and efforts to provide a service to meet the needs of women, at present unrecognised by existing provision.

I and many others feel, that the ability of women to influence their health care lies in their unity around that common cause, cutting across the class and racial boundaries; it would be extremely naive, however, if we failed to acknowledge that these exist, for it would mean that we had failed to realise that while women share common problems, their perceptions and experience of these differ. Our collective efforts in self-help and self-education will increase our own awareness and understanding of each other's needs and expectations, and the barriers, both social and economic, to achieving these.

A well woman conference was held in March 1985, at which it was agreed by the women present that there was a need for a Women's Health Information and Support Centre (WHISC). Interest was also expressed in a women's health training course, the aim of which was to help women develop their self-confidence and skills, in counselling, the promotion of health education and a positive attitude to health care. The skills developed by women attending the course would provide the basis for setting up a centre that would provide a place where women could meet informally to discuss their problems, get information (not medical advice) on how they may best be dealt with and where to go for further information and advice. It would also act as a community resource whereby the women staffing the centre would encourage and help women within the community to set up their own localised self-help health groups. This liaison would also enable information from the local groups to be channelled back to the centre, so that it would continue to evolve and be responsive to women's needs.

Thus far, we have set up a working party to plan and pursue funding, and so on, for a mobile service in the form of a women's health bus, with the long-term objective of a possible permanent site. A mobile health promotion service has just been launched by South Sefton Area Health Authority and we are watching this imaginative initiative with hope and interest.

The first 12-week course has almost finished and it is hoped that the group will remain in being and meet regularly and, perhaps, invite speakers to their meetings.

The course offers 10 counselling sessions geared to developing basic skills in listening and communication, with group discussion, videos and speakers on a wide variety of topics, eg. depression, premenstrual tension, and child sexual abuse. The information given is also slanted toward use in developing self-help groups and the promotion of health education. Those attending the course are self-selected on the basis of their commitment to women's health, and no formal qualifications are required. The emphasis is on the sharing of experiences, skills and knowledge and encouraging the development of women's self confidence. A number of women from the course, in particular those from the black community, have offered their time and set up a temporary base at the Vauxhall Community Centre, their efforts being centred on speeding up the achievement of our common objective: these are much appreciated by us all. We remain optimistic about achieving our goal, and the future benefits of this to the community.

For me, these six months have been most interesting and worthwhile. As someone who has previously worked as a health professional, I feel that these community initiatives are both an imaginative and practical approach to health education and preventive health care. Whilst lay health workers may be seen by some as a threat to the health professionals, my personal feeling is that they should be actively encouraged for a number of reasons. Firstly, whilst I acknowledge the major benefits derived from the NHS, one cannot deny that major health and health care inequalities still exist, and in the light of present cutbacks, these could be exacerbated. For a number of reasons, certain social groups are less likely to take up the services available. It is all too easy to resort to 'victim blaming' to explain this, particularly when one considers the criticisms levelled at the service by those who do use it. I would suggest that those active in the community may be in a better position to provide information on local needs and expectations.

Secondly, there are many within the NHS who are sensitive to consumer needs and demands, but, like the consumer, find it difficult to effect change, given the bureaucratic and hierarchical structure of the service. Whilst the pursuit of professionalism can be understood with regard to standards of care, pay and working conditions, it could prove detrimental to the consumers and professionals in the long term. Professionalism, the control of knowledge and practice, whilst protecting the interests of consumers and health professionals, can have a double edge. The insularity, inward looking attitudes and protective mechanisms generated by professionals may serve to reinforce inequalities in health and health care. As they tend to see health in their terms, this may make them less responsive to criticism, in order to protect that model of health and health care. Hence, I welcome the proposed educational changes which seek to place nurse-education within Colleges of Further

Education because the student may develop a less restricted view of health and a more adaptable and flexible approach to health care. Within this context, lay health workers and women's self-help groups within the community, may be seen to facilitate the development of health education and preventive health care. The links established with those sympathetic and committed professionals may be seen eventually as providing better channels of communication and understanding between the professionals and consumers.

The dialogue established will enable the consumer to understand the constraints imposed on health professionals and the professionals to be more responsive to the community's health needs. It will, one hopes, provide the framework by which health professionals and lay workers based in the community can together provide an imaginative approach to health and health care. Our objectives are the same and the means of achieving this should not be seen as encroaching on the health professionals' territory, but rather as a way of facilitating a collective approach to the problems which bedevil us all.

Health, in the widest sense of the word, should be seen as a person's birthright. In a wealthy industrial society this should be seen also as a major objective to be pursued both imaginatively and collectively on the basis of shared knowledge, skills and experience.

In pursuit of this ideal I wish to acknowledge particularly the vision and unflagging efforts of Libby and Margaret, who, supported by the Vauxhall Neighbourhood Council, initiated an imaginative approach to community health. Also Merseyside County Council Women's Interest Committee, and all the women and men, both black and white, too numerous to name, who continue to offer practical help and support in the continuing development of this approach to health care.

Chapter 11
ECONOMIC ASPECTS OF WOMEN'S HEALTH

Wendy Hull

A Model of decision-making: a simple application

Today is pay day, the money's in the bank or the cash is in your pocket . . . and hard earned it has been this week. Walking home, a jacket in a shop window attracts your attention. Trying it on, it fits well and you feel good wearing it. It would be just right for this chilly Spring weather and, more importantly, it could be worn over your blue dress to make an outfit smart enough for Cousin Jean's wedding – what a saving that would be! In your mind, these 'innumerable' benefits that you will derive from having the jacket in your wardrobe more than offset the cost. The decision's made, the jacket is purchased.

A familiar enough sequence, a decision that you would not expect to ponder further – you feel perfectly justified in spending your own hard-earned money in any way that you wish and obviously do not expect to have to defend your ranking of the benefits derived from ownership to anyone.

We see in this simple illustration, the essence of decision-making: each individual has a valuing system that converts (in this case) the cost of the jacket, measured in monetary terms, into the benefits derived from owning it. The jacket makes you feel good, it matches other items in your wardrobe, so it will be worn often, and perhaps will save further cash outlay on an outfit for the wedding. None of these benefits can be easily expressed in monetary terms, but in your valuing system, they add up to more than the price tag on the jacket.

Decision-making with public funds

Quite rightly, our simple illustration should be dismissed: it is but one of a number of such decisions that we expect to make daily. Having earned the cash, it is an individual's right to spend it in any way that maximises the benefits to that individual.

Let us now consider an equally familiar situation, but this time the cash we are spending is not our own but public funds. While driving to the office, the health visitor contemplates the coming day. Thursday, Baby Clinic this afternoon 2–4 pm. Good, I can collect the breast pump from the clinic and deliver it afterwards to Mrs Green. Hopefully that will help her to maintain breast feeding, she's already feeling depressed and inadequate in her ability to cope with her baby daughter; being unable to continue breast feeding would be the final straw. While I'm in Mrs Green's road, I can call round the corner and check why Mrs Black didn't bring her toddler for his immunisation appointment.

Now . . . this morning, I must get back to Mrs Grey, she's feeling very guilty about her mother's transfer to a nursing home. What else can she do with three little ones to look after? Then I must see the two new babies on the patch, both ten days old today. By the time I've got back, done the notes and picked up the dry-cleaning, the morning will be gone. That means that I probably won't be able to pop in on Mrs White today for the baby's six months assessment, but that can wait a few more days.

Again, the sort of planning and decision-making that preceeds the typical day of a busy health visitor. Decision-making that is assumed to be effective in achieving its objective of making the most of the working day, a skill that she has, of necessity, developed to cope with the many demands made on her time.

In contrast to our simple example, the health visitor's resources are not directly measured in money terms. The resource that she will be spending in the course of the day is a given number of skilled and trained HV hours. The pay cheque puts a value on those hours at the current salary scale. But in deciding how best to use her time, the health visitor is weighing up the demands on her against the amount of time she has available that day.

So, from the way in which the health visitor plans her day, what can we learn about how she intends to spend the resources at her disposal? Some of her time has been predetermined: the Baby Clinic is a set weekly event. So in a sense, the community wants, in exchange for the cost of a health visitor, a regular Baby Clinic with a health visitor present. Similarly, the visits to the two 10-day old infants, being a statutory requirement, reflect an assumption on society's part that the benefits of such visits are worth the cost of paying the health visitor to make them. In terms of our earlier decision-making model, the benefits derived by the community in general from baby clinics and 10-day visiting must be adjudged to exceed the costs of providing those services otherwise, presumably, the provision of those services could no longer be justified.

What about the remainder of the health visitor's day? On closer examination we see her making similar trade-offs between alternative ways of using her time in order to provide the best service to her patients. The benefit of getting the breast pump to Mrs Green was expressed in terms of trying to relieve some of the patient's problems of anxiety and depression. The cost of Mrs Green being unable to cope is such that she ranks as being the most important visit to make after the Baby Clinic. Certainly, the benefits of visiting Mrs Green are judged by the health visitor to exceed those derived from visiting Mrs White. The assessment visit to Mrs White can be deferred: the resources (HV hours) have already been spent in providing services perceived to derive greater benefits.

An explicit statement of this trading-off by the health visitor runs along the lines that Mrs Green is in danger of needing hospitalisation should her depression increase. Costs will be associated with that in terms of both inpatient care and the cost to the family of another relative having to stay at home and look after the toddler and Grandma, who is not too well. A deferrment of Mrs White's assessment visit is not anticipated to produce such costly knock-on effects.

The parallels with the simple decision on the jacket should be apparent. In both situations resources were spent (cash for the jacket and HV hours) in exchange for benefits that could not be so easily quantified. The benefits derived are valued by each of us, not in money terms, but according to our own individual scales of preference. The value of feeling good in the jacket can never be quantified, nor should time be spent in trying to do so. In buying the jacket, your own scale of values needs no justifying – you were spending your own cash. But the health visitor was making similar judgements about the benefits derived from spending her time on certain visits, assuming that the visits she made gave the greatest return and postponing those that she considered to be less effective that day.

Again, it is quite right and proper that this is a fair responsibility given to professionals such as health visitors. From understanding their role in the community they are effectively equipped to so plan and structure their working day. But the important ingredient to recognise is that each health visitor has her own valuing system and uses it to rank priorities: public funds are then committed against that ranking. Arguably, every health professional should reflect occasionally on her own assumptions about benefits derived from different courses of action. Why did Mrs Green rank above Mrs White? Surely Mrs Black was not the only mother to miss an immunisation appointment? What is it about the value of the benefits derived from visiting her that make her a more pressing priority amongst all the others? If we cannot measure directly the benefits of making the visit, we tend to think in terms of what would be the cost of not making the visit. So the opportunity cost of visiting Mrs Green is equivalent to the possible hospitalisation and domestic help costs avoided by maintaining her at home. In this case, the opportunity cost is defined as the cost of next best alternative avoided.

PLANNING HEALTH CARE SERVICES – THE DECISION

Let us now move decision-making into a wider dimension and consider the provision of all health care services within the community as a whole, and not just one health visitor on a patch in Manchester (or wherever).

The nature of society at present is such that the resources available to provide health care services are limited: usually, they are considered to be limited in terms of money. The Government, supposedly reflecting the people's wishes, is only prepared to make 'so much' available for the health services at any given point of time. Even if that constraint were lifted, however, unlimited health care would not be available as we have only 'so many' doctors, nurses and other health professionals trained and available to provide services in the short/medium term. So, as with the simple example of the jacket, where total resources were limited to the size of the pay packet, and that of the health visitor on her rounds where the total resources available to 'spend' were the hours in her working day, the total resources available for health care as a whole are similarily limited.

The parallels with the earlier examples continue. In deciding how best to spend our total health care resources we must make some judgements about the benefits derived from providing a certain mix of services as against any of the innumerable alternative combinations of services. The health visitor had any number of people that she could consider visiting on that day, but she planned her day around those few individuals who she judged would most benefit from a visit that day: she was able to carry in her head all the information needed to rank those alternatives.

Can every health care planner put hand on heart and make the same claim about the current provision of health care to the general community? Inevitably, our current pattern of health services is not necessarily that which provides the best combination of services to those in need – it still largely reflects historical influences. Ideally, we should be able to say that our health services commit the limited resources available in such a way as to maximise the benefits to the community in need as a whole. Furthermore, the community in need is not a collection of homogeneous individuals. Instead, it comprises men and women, boys and girls, newborn infants and ageing grandparents. Middle-aged working men suffering from ulcers, bronchitis and heart attacks and their middle-aged wives with elderly mothers to care for, newly-married and pregnant daughters needing moral support and advice and a teenage son threatening a nervous collapse over his A levels.

How do we ensure that the competing claims of all these equally legitimate health care groups are met in equal measures, given that we do not have unlimited resources to commit against their demands for services. Do health care planners see these groups as having equal claims to resources? Or do we detect in their decision-making an implicit ranking of the desirability of spending money on one group in preference to some other? Does the pattern of services as currently provided put a greater value on, for instance, intensive care for the newborn against day care provision for the elderly mentally infirm. Is it more 'beneficial' to provide health care services for the employed population rather than dependants such as wives not employed outside the home? How do we begin to bring rationality into such difficult decisions?

Cost effectiveness

Health care services are frequently justified in terms of their cost-effectiveness. Essentially, the phrase embodies the same approach to decision-making as we have already explored, namely that expenditure is committed when the resultant benefits are expected to exceed those costs. The greater the benefits relative to the costs of providing the service, the more cost-effective the service is said to be.

A good example of a generally accepted cost-effective service is the immunisation programme for pre- and school-age children. The benefits in terms of the virtual elimination of diseases such as diptheria, tetanus and poliomyelitis greatly exceed the costs involved in immunising the children. More recently, though, we have learnt that the equation is less simple for whooping cough. A reduced incidence of the disease is bought not just at the cost of the actual immunisation procedure but also at the cost of several cases of vaccine-damaged children. At what point do we consider any benefits to be outweighed by the costs? 10 vaccine-damaged children? 100 or 1000 such handicapped children? In making that trade-off, exactly how are we measuring the cost of a vaccine-damaged child? In terms of the suffering of the child and its parents – presumably beyond measurement? In a more detached way by considering the cost of state care for the handicapped child?

Again, we see at the heart of decision-making a need to place a value on benefits. We want to spend our limited health care resources on cost-effective services, but what does this classification mean when we have no currency with which to measure effectiveness for comparison with cost. Whooping cough vaccination for most of us would rank as an effective service, but not in the valuing system of the relatives of children handicapped as a result. We talk easily of 'effectiveness' but what or whose underlying ranking of preferences is implicit in the classification?

Cost-benefit analysis and option appraisal

In more recent times, economists have attempted to model decision-making in such a way as to make the underlying assumptions explicit and quantifiable. The technique is called cost-benefit analysis. (Summaries can be found in Frost 1971; Kendal 1971.)

Cost-benefit analysis (CBA) attempts to measure the social costs and benefits of a plan in monetary values. We have already identified that the tangible costs and benefits of any proposal are usually comparatively easy to forecast and express in cash terms. Our previous examples of decision-making ran into problems trying to quantify the variety of rather more nebulous aspects of the decision.

CBA was first applied in the USA in the 1930s and in the UK in the 1950s, when it was applied to the project to build the M1 motorway. The decision concerning the third London Airport continues to be a well-publicised more recent application. To understand the technique consider the decision to install overhead lighting on the M1 motorway between Newport Pagnall and London. The effectiveness of such lighting is recognised to be significant in reducing road traffic accidents. Accidents involve costs to the community including caring for the injured, perhaps in hospital, the loss of earnings whilst they are off work, as well as the emotional cost to the individuals and to the remainder of the families who have to cope.

Even the enormous costs of installing and maintaining neon lighting along 40 miles of the motorway could be justified if true weight were given to the social benefits mentioned. The process of measuring intangible benefits forces the planners to make explicit the anticipated social consequences of their decision. The expression of those social consequences in financial terms exposes the planners underlying values. For instance, we in this society value an individual life very highly and consequently vast project costs, as in this case, can be justified in terms of 'savings' through road accident deaths avoided. Important though the technique is, CBA still tends to be limited to major government schemes because the studies themselves involve costs and need experienced staff. The problems associated with the identification and measurement of social costs and benefits are real and great. A more useful and simpler application of the technique more suited to the needs of the health care planner is option appraisal.

Option appraisal, like CBA, is concerned with the need to lay bare the implicit valuing or preference system used when comparing the costs and benefits of any decision. CBA exposes those assumptions by expressing them in financial terms, option appraisal is rather more subtle. At the core of any decision is the analysis of how will the desired objectives be best achieved. Option appraisal elicits from decision-makers the ranking of project proposals in terms of how well each achieves the agreed desired objectives (or desiderata). The need to provide detailed financial information is avoided but the decision on which option to adopt has been made with reference to objective data rather than the decision-makers preferences or intuitions.

So the requirement of CBA to quantify in absolute terms such costs as a life lost or impaired in a motorway accident is replaced in option appraisal by the need to rank in relative terms costs and benefits associated with particular decisions. Specifically, is one life saved by a heart transplant valued more highly than the enhancement of several lives through minor surgery purchased at the same cost? Ranking in relative terms such vastly different ways of spending the same cash makes explicit the decision-makers preferences. The existence of preferences is unavoidable, the opportunity to examine and agree with or dispute those preferences is rarely offered.

It is because resources to spend on health care are limited in total that health care planning necessarily involves choices; one service (heart transplants, in our previous example) is provided at the expense of another (minor surgery) – both cannot be afforded. What such a decision actually involves is the ranking of the 'value' of the benefit to the heart disease sufferer relative to the 'value' to the several, say, varicose vein sufferers. Any such ranking decisions involve implicit assumptions about the relative worth of the various members of the community. Do we, or should we, value a premature infant's life more highly than that of its aged, mentally-infirm grandmother? Do we feel that a given sum of money is 'better spent' on neonatal care than on psychogeriatrics? Health-care planning cannot avoid such difficult decisions. Sadly, planners often avoid making explicit their underlying valuing assumptions, preferring to give in to what are 'politically acceptable' preferences.

With this theoretical background we can now explore what the pattern of health care services for women tells us about the value placed on women by society.

THE VALUE OF HEALTH CARE SERVICES FOR WOMEN

The policy underlying health care provision is to undertake investment in cost effective services. The services provided are justified in terms of giving greatest benefit to patients relative to costs. But, as we have seen, benefits cannot be simply and objectively quantified in £s; their 'value' derives from personal preferences and attitudes. Ideally, the pattern of health care services should reflect the collective preferences of the community served and policy-makers should adopt techniques that make explicit the priorities that has been assumed.

Successful or effective services are often so measured in terms of 'cures', or 'positives' if a screening programme. Such simple criteria might be appropriate if it were equally legitimate to give the same value to all members of the community. We do not in fact do this: for instance, it is often assumed, that the best interests of society are served by providing services to maintain the 'working population' at work; after all, is it not on these productive members that we all depend economically? What, however, does such a statement tell us about the implicit value attached to one such member of the community relative to say a retired man, or a woman working in the home rather than for an employer. Let us explore the issue from a different direction. A leading medical journal recently published the results of an eight-year Swedish study involving more than 130,000 women that offered all but conclusive evidence that X-ray screening or mammography can cut the death-rate from breast cancer amongst older women (Tabar 1985). In a leading article the journal states that there is no longer much dispute that early detection and treatment can alter the course of the disease. The new survey also confirms other findings that mammography is more effective than clinical examination. About 20,000 women a year develop breast cancer with 12,600 dying in 1983: early diagnosis reduces the liklihood of the cancer cells spreading to other parts of the body and increases the possibility of a cure.

On the strength of this evidence, it is suggested that women at risk identified from the records of local Family Practitioner Committees should be invited for screening on the basis 'that the Government will provide additional funds for this life-saving cause, rather than expecting health authorities to divert resources from areas of pressing need'. If the examination is so effective and potentially life-saving, why doesn't the service go immediately to the top of the priority list? With such conclusive evidence, should we not be diverting resources from some less effective service in order to provide breast mammography? By failing to do that, how are we actually valuing the lives of the 12,600 women who died of breast cancer in 1983? Logically, the policy-makers should continually be reviewing the current pattern of services and asking whether the benefits of the present services outweigh the benefits of spending the same cash on the provision of breast cancer mammography. The reality is that the X-ray department can only cope with so many investigations each day. Physical resources such as the number of machines and trained staff are limited in the short/medium term. So which investigations should be stopped in order to undertake mammorgaphy? Fractures? Barium meals? Ultrasound scans? Cardiac investigations?

There are no easy answers. But some objectivity could be introduced by explicitly ranking the value of a woman's life lost through breast cancer against say a man's life lost from a heart attack or that of a baby with congenital problems. If as a consequence we actually believe that the resources of the X-ray department cannot be more effectively used, fine. Mammography cannot be justified, we have demonstrated that the benefits to other groups of patients are greater. To avoid this central issue and divert attention towards a general cry for more resources suggests that the need to save deaths from breast cancer is not a sufficiently pressing need that it takes priority over the existing pattern of services. Furthermore, any such argument entirely neglects the point that money spent on preventive screening should be justified in terms of treatment costs avoided through early detection.

As if this weren't enough, women's services seem to be under attack from an additional direction: on the one hand, there seem to be real problems associated with new screening programmes as we have just been examining, while on the other, a question-mark perpetually hangs over the 'effectiveness' of existing services. Arguments rage about the viability of cervical screening programmes: Few 'positives' seem to be identified relative to the considerable costs of the computerised recall system for women at risk. A low pick-up rate is often quoted as evidence of an ineffective service that should be curtailed and the resources diverted elsewhere. Again, this reasoning has failed to recognise that the cost of the screening programme may be more than justified if we realistically measure the true 'worth' of the lives of those women identified as 'positives'.

As discussed, one approach is to think in terms of the cost of replacing the contribution made by a woman who dies of undetected cervical cancer. What is the cost to society of alternative care for the children, support for the husband, the cost of hospitalising the elderly relative living with the family and nursed by the wife, and the cost of some other means of support for the disabled neighbour next door? The network of care and support that is so often the daily routine of many 'non-working' wives is extensive and so very often quite taken for granted until the day when the wife is herself ill and the whole collapses. Although a woman's contribution cannot be conveniently measured in terms of working days lost, any such superficial examination suggests that her value is enormous.

To some, cervical cytology is virtually synomous with a well woman clinic. To attempt to evaluate the success of well woman clinics with a single and simple criterion such as percentage of positive smears identified is a nonsense. As earlier chapters amply demonstrate, well woman clinics are the ideal setting for the early detection of so many health problems: they are undoubtedly cost effective if a true measure of the contribution of women to the community is built into the benefits side of the equation.

The only realistic approach to quantifying the benefits of preventive services is in terms of the costs that prevention avoids. Early detection and treatment of breast cancer, as we saw, can save costs associated with more radical operative procedures required after later detection. The well woman clinics aim to teach health awareness, give dietary and healthy living advice, effective contraceptive guidance, and generally address health issues of importance to women. In the short term, spending on such services may seem to be giving a poor return and it is difficult to justify the expenditure against competing claims. The understanding and application of the economic considerations explored in this chapter should help in arguments for a greater share of limited resources. Specifically, the value of women in terms of their opportunity cost should be recognised. If money is not spent on preventive services for women, then the community must realise that there is a cost to replacing the services of women who subsequently become ill. Simple expressions of cost effectiveness are inadequate if they fail to accept that cost cannot be easily equated with 'cures'. Costs can be justified if we give true recognition to the contribution made by women and decision-makers are forced to make explicit the value they place on that contribution.

Concluding considerations

Other chapters in this book ably make the case for, and demonstrate the benefits of, well woman clinics. Increasingly today, questions are being directed against expensive, high-technology medicine that is committed to a predominantly curative approach. Under such a regime, many of the patients' true problems are either not expressed or are ignored, misunderstood or dismissed. Women need time to talk and express their fears and problems to another women (generally a doctor or health visitor). Added to this, the women's movement seeks to establish that every woman has a right to their own bodies. The well woman clinic provides a model that undeniably fills this widening gap in health care services.

Committed to this ideal, the health care professional can marshall a range of arguments to support the setting up of such a service, only to be frustrated by inability to secure even modest funds for implementation. At this point, the relevance of this brief excursion into economic thinking should become apparent. Having gained a true understanding of the concepts outlined in this chapter, the health professional should be able to make an irrefutable case for funding to even the most parsimonious of treasurers.

As already discussed, it is wholly correct that in order to secure funding, a service should demonstrate cost effectiveness: that is, the benefits derived from the service should outweigh the costs of providing the service. The assessment and scheduling of the costs of proposed service appears straightforward. Staff time required at different grades can be calculated at current rates of pay, plus various on-costs for National Insurance and Superannuation. Accommodation costs will be known from experience of heating, lighting and rating similar properties. An examination of the cost of running other patient services and discussion with the health personnel involved will give a good indication of the sums of money required for equipment, comsumables and other such items. But, all too often neglected is the 'benefits' side of the equation. The justification of funds for any service, including well woman clinics, is in demonstrating that real and quantifiable benefits accrue that are cost-saving or cost-preventing to the health services as a whole.

In this respect, consider the contribution to the community made by women on a true opportunity-cost basis – what is the true cost to society of women's undetected health problems? What does it cost the community to replace the services to the family no longer provided by a woman because of ill health or premature death? Yet further savings will be made in other health and social services as a result of improved health knowledge and awareness learned at the well woman clinic. A modest spending on promotion of healthy living now must outweigh the long-term cost of continuing physical and/or mental ill health. Expressed in true economic terms, with due recognition of the cost to society of trying to replace the services rendered to the community by women, this should make the financial argument for well woman clinics overwhelming. Against the schedule of direct financial costs of implementing such a service, work needs to be undertaken to consider quantifying the following factors:

- the size of the target population
- the current pattern of the use of GP and hospital services by this population
- the current birth rate and the nature of, and spending on, maternity and children's services
- quantify the savings through good contraceptive services provided for and sought by a wider section of women
- quantify the savings through improved diet and healthier living for the whole family

- quantify the effect of reduced use of GP and hospital services from earlier disease detection and wider health promotion

Admittedly, tackling such concepts is far more difficult than scheduling costs which can be precisely calculated, but unless some sensible attempts are made to measure the benefits that instinctively all committed to well woman clinics recognise, it will increasingly be all too easy to dismiss the idea as failing in cost-effectiveness.

Further reading

Readers interested in developing the ideas introduced in this chapter are referred to the following suggested texts:

Algie J (1983) Everything you wanted to know about priority scaling. *Health and Social Services Journal*, November, 1320–1321

Frost M J (1971) *Values for Money. The Technique of Cost Benefit Analysis*. London: Gower

Jones R & Pendlebury M (1984) *Public Sector Accounting*. London: Pitman

Jones T & Prowle M (1984) *Health Service Finance*. Certified Accountants Educational Trust

Kendal M G (1971) *Cost Benefit Analysis*. London: English Universities Press

Layard R (1972) *Cost Benefit Analysis*. Harmondsworth: Penguin Books

Misham E J (1976) *Elements of Cost Benefit Analysis*. London: Allen & Unwin

Sullivan C & Adair R (1984) Project appraisal in the public sector. *Public Finance and Accountancy*, March, 28–29

Tabar I (1985) Reduction in mortality from breast cancer after breast screening with mammography. *Lancet*, April 13, 829–832

IN CONCLUSION

Jean Orr

We have now considered some of the theoretical issues related to women's health and examined how different groups of workers in the North West of England have provided services to meet local need. In many communities there is a discernible trend which is cutting across class and political groupings – the spontaneous ad hoc organisation of women to meet a particular need or to combine against a specific threat. This is evident in the range of self-help and protest groups which have mushroomed in the last 5–10 years, examples being the Rape Crisis Centres and Women's Aid, as well as well woman groups and centres.

This should come as no surprise to those of us who recognise that the matters women most care about, and are responsible for, happen at home, in the community. This differs from the world of most men for whom the core of their life is work and the activities associated with it. Women are very aware that the community they inhabit is not the community idealised by politicians but it is the place where women are in direct contact and confrontation with the State as represented by housing, welfare and health services. For many women their contacts with these services only reinforce their roles and make implicit and explicit the degree of their failure.

Many of the early community development schemes ignored women's problems and criticism of the treatment of women's issues has grown. Mayo (1977) saw that there was a tendency to reinforce sexist role stereotyping by concentrating on women as wives and mothers, thus failing to facilitate the developments of other facets of their personalities or meet other needs and aspirations. Health visitors and nurses still place insufficient emphasis on the community specifically as it effects women.

Many health visitors are involved in organising mother and toddler groups but it could be argued that the function of these groups is little more than a reflection of middle class values and views of women. Health visitors may therefore not be involved in consciousness raising or in encouraging action to ameliorate neglected issues such as the health problems of older women. For example, it was not health care professionals who actively campaigned for refuges for women who are abused. Indeed, it could be argued that the professionals have been prepared to ignore issues of violence against women because it disturbs the accepted view and values of family life. The fact that women themselves are organising is indicative of their concern and their determination to effect change. The women's health movement is a good example of how women have challenged the health care professionals and have spearheaded a nation-wide movement.

To work with women in the community we have to be prepared to change much of the existing client/professional relationship and means of service delivery. There are many innovatory schemes operating throughout the UK, some of which are described in the Report of the Working Group on Women and the Health Service (WNC 1984). There is no doubt that women are a major force in the community health movement which, according to Rosenthal (1983), is a growing and a distinct part of health provision in Britain. This movement is said to be based outside the health professionals and concerned with inequalities in health and health care provision. It is based on the belief that the achievement of a healthy community depends on a collective awareness of the social causes of ill health and positive health and is concerned to challenge at an individual and collective level the monopoly of information about health and ill health by health professionals.

How are we to respond to this community health movement? Rebekah Williams has discussed the strengths and difficulties when professionals and lay workers are working together. As professionals we have to recognise that the powerful professional approach is inappropriate. The interaction has to be one of equals with lay workers and the women using the services. This is the approach of the Child Development Programme which is a large-scale health visiting intervention programme with disadvantage families (Orr 1985). We have the evidence that women want a different range of services and we have to decide how we can best meet their needs. We can no longer assume traditional services are appropriate or that we are 'doing it anyway'.

For example, a local women's health group in Manchester organised a series of six talks on health issues such as depression, diet and stress, the average attendance at which was between 50–70 each evening. At the same time, local health visitors were saying that there was no need for these talks and that they would not be well attended. They were sadly out of touch, and I suspect they are not alone. Women are interested in themselves and will seek advice if it is offered in a form which they understand. It may be that too many have only experienced NHS groups in mothercraft or parentcraft classes which are often solely geared to professionals goals and are out of touch with the concerns of pregnant women. It is indicative of the importance placed on these classes that we see them as an opportunity for a range of nurses to practice teaching skills: it says a lot about how we view the status of women. I doubt if we would send students to talk to groups of men at the local Institute of Marketing or the Round Table: we would not dare to devalue them in this way.

According to Goeppinger *et al.* (1982), community health nurses should assist communities to recognise and meet their collective needs. They do this by identifying problems and assets in the community and intervening to strengthen the interactions within the community. This approach can be described as working with the collectivity as a unit and is different from working with the constituent parts of that unit; in other words, the individuals and families. It is a common assumption to equate delivering health care to individuals and families who happen to live in the community, with working at a community level with community health issues. However, operating at a community level means working with various groups and networks, not concentrating only on individuals and families. This type of work is based on the belief that women have the capacity to join together and take action on their own behalf and that the provision of services is more likely to be taken up if they are geared to the needs and priorities articulated by local women as Effie Sherlock shows. Nurses must therefore help women to develop the skills of collective activity and the skills of decision making. They must also help in the development of local groups.

There is little evidence that we can be complaisant about the development of new services for women or, indeed, certain that existing services will continue. As Clare Ronalds and Merryn Cooke point out, it is not simply enough to have good ideas and committed workers; there needs to be commitment from managers who control budgets. Both Joan Armstrong and Rebekah Williams show that consumer satisfaction alone may not be enough to overcome NHS institutional arthritis and professional jealousies. Wendy Hull makes it clear that economic decisions are not separate from the dominant values of system in society, a value system which is male-dominated. What seems evident is the possibility of a backlash and retrenchment on women health provision. The issues about women controlling their bodies and health has been explored in many of the chapters. It is crucial that we hold on to what freedom and choices we have both for ourselves and our clients. We know that as resources become scarce well woman services will be increasingly under threat, despite the fact that the clinics described here fulfil much of the rhetoric of the WHO view of primary health care. Our clinics are

(a) concerned with prevention;
(b) meeting local and articulated needs;
(c) involving local communities and forming partnerships;
(d) using voluntary helpers;
(e) based on a self help ethos;
(f) reaching clients not covered by existing services; and
(g) bringing together a range of disciplines and looking at the whole person.

The holistic approach to health care refers to a qualitatively different approach, one that respects the interaction of mind, body and environment. Ferguson (1982) describes the assumption of the holistic approach and this is similar to the philosophy of well woman clinics.

Holistic care is said, among other things, to
- be concerned with the whole person;
- see the person as autonomous; and
- Depend primarily on qualitative information incuding the person's subjective reports and professionals' intuition.

The women's health movement owes its existence to the reemergence of feminism. Feminist analysis of society has enabled us to see that women suffer from structural inequalities in society based on sex as well as class.

The feminist literature has also provided us with substantive material on women's health and women's lives which should form an important part of nursing, midwifery and health visiting education (Orr 1986). At present, little is taught which is particularly relevant to women and much of the social sciences are, in fact, grounded in and derived from the experiences, perceptions and beliefs of men (Evans 1983).

Feminists have shown that there is no psychology, no sociology, no anthropology of women. The problems and priorities of women are regarded as unimportant and main areas of women's lives such as childbirth and sexuality have only been examined if they pose problems for the male world. Because men control language we have no words to name what we experience (Spender 1980). What positive words do we have to name the rich and varied feelings of motherhood, birthing or menstruation? The work of feminist writers raises questions for us as nurses about how much we should be involved in helping women validate their own experience as opposed to helping to perpetuate essentially male values and meanings. Can we share the hopes of Adrienne Rich (1977) that woman should be the presiding genius of her own body?

I believe we can move some way towards that goal by utilising the existing substantive material on women's lives and women's health to inform practice and education. This requires a critical examination of what happens in education and a recognition of the values and beliefs which underpin much of existing practice. Most urgently, we need to change the nature of the relationship between ourselves and women by moving to a more equal model and giving power and control to those we seek to help. The women's health movement is one way forward.

Reference

Evans M (1983) In praise of theory. The case for women's studies. In Bowles G & Duelli Klein R (eds) *Theories of Women's Studies*. London: Routlege & Kegan Paul

Ferguson M (1982) *The Aquarian Conspiracy Personal and Social Transformation in the 1980s*. London: Granada

Goeppinger J, Lassiter P & Wilcox B (1982) Community Health in community competence. *Nursing Outlook.* **30** (8), 464–467

Mayo M (1977) *Women in the Community.* London: Routledge & Kegan Paul

Orr J (1985) Assessing Family and individuals. In Luker K & Orr J (eds) *Health Visiting.* Oxford: Blackwell Scientific Publications

Orr J (1986) Feminism and health visiting. In Webb C (ed) *Feminist Practice in Women's Health Care.* Chichester: Wiley/ HM & M

Rich A (1977) *Off Women Born.* London: Virago

Rosenthal M (1983) Neighbourhood Health Projects. *Community Development Journal,* **18** (2), 120–131

Spender D (1980) *Man Made Language.* London: Routledge & Kegan Paul

Womens National Campaign (1984) *Working Group on Women and Health Services.* London: Cabinet Offices

Appendix

WELL WOMAN CLINIC QUESTIONNAIRE

This example of a Well Woman Clinic Questionnaire is reproduced by courtesy of South Manchester Health Authority. It is set out here in an abbreviated format – more space than that shown will be needed for the answers to some of the questions.

SOUTH MANCHESTER HEALTH AUTHORITY
COMMUNITY HEALTH SERVICES

CONFIDENTIAL

WELL WOMEN CLINIC – YOU AND YOUR HEALTH

WORKER	No. ....
NURSE	DATE ....
DOCTOR	AGE ....

HEALTH PROFILE

Have you come mainly for a general check-up or for any special reason?	YES, Check-up	YES, reason
If you came for a special reason, have you seen anyone else about this?	YES WHO?	NO

If you have, what did they say?

Are you taking any medicine (including sleeping pills) or being treated for anything at present?	YES	NO	

If YES, details please

Medicines	For What?	From Whom?

Do you get headaches? DETAILS	YES	NO	
Any trouble with eyes or vision? DETAILS	YES	NO	
Any trouble with teeth? DETAILS	YES	NO	
Any trouble with hearing? DETAILS	YES	NO	
Do you have a cough? DETAILS	YES	NO	
Do you examine your breasts regularly?	YES	NO	SOME-TIMES
Would yoy like to learn?	YES	NO	
Do you suffer from indigestion? DETAILS	YES	NO	

| Do you have a good appetite? | YES | NO |
DETAILS

| Do you have problems with | YES | NO |
DETAILS

Do you get repeated cystitis?

YES
NO
DETAILS

LAST MENSTRUAL PERIOD
Have you had any problems with your period or your menstrual cycle?
| YES | NO | DETAILS: |

Have you any problems to do with the menopause (the change)?
| YES | NO | DETAILS: |

Do you use any method of contraception?
| YES | NO | WHICH METHOD: |

Any problems with it?
| YES | NO | DETAILS: |

Have you ever wanted a baby, but had difficulty in getting pregnant?
| YES | NO | DETAILS: |

| Have you got a vaginal discharge: | YES | NO |

Can you describe it?
DETAILS

| Does it bother you? | YES | NO |
DETAILS:

Have you ever had a cervical smear?	YES	NO	DON'T KNOW

If YES, when was the last one?
Do you know what the result was?

Any trouble with piles?	YES	NO

DETAILS:

Any trouble with varicose veins?	YES	NO

DETAILS:

Any trouble with feet?

YES
NO
DETAILS:

Do you have any other worries about your physical health?	YES	NO

If YES, what?

Lots of things influence how healthy we feel, and we would like to ask you about some of them now.

YOU AND YOUR HEALTH

Who else lives in your household?

Relationship	Age	What to they do (job)	Have they changed their job recently?

Anyone else in the family who doesn't live with you?

How long have you been at your present address?

Have you any housing problems?
YES   NO   DETAILS

Have you any financial problems?
YES   NO   DETAILS

Have you suffered any bereavements lately?
YES   NO   DETAILS

Do you have anyone to help you out if you need it?
YES   NO   DETAILS

Do you have anyone who you can talk over your probems with and confide in?
YES   NO   DETAILS

Do you ever feel isolated and lonely?
YES   NO   DETAILS

Are you working at the moment?   YES   NO

How do you feel about it?

Do you have much time off work   YES   NO

Have you any problems connected with work?   YES   NO

YOUR LIFESTYLE AND FEELINGS

Smoking

Do you smoke?
(Please give details)

Do you want to give up?

Have you tried to give up?

Drinking
Do you like a drink (alcohol)
About how much do you drink?

Eating
What did you eat
yesterday for: BREAKFAST..
              MID-DAY ....
              EVENING ....

What else did you have?
(including alcohol)

Was this typical? (if not, what is)?

How much to you weigh?　　　　　　Height:

Are you happy about your weight?
YES　　　　　　NO
If NO, why not?　　　　　DETAILS:

Has there been much change in your weight over the last year?
YES　　　　　　NO　　　　　　DETAILS:

Would you like any advice about diet?
YES　　　　　　NO　　　　　　DETIALS:

Enjoying Life
Do you have any time for yourself?
YES　　　　　　NO　　　　　　DETAILS:

Are you content with the way you spend your free time?
YES　　　　　　NO　　　　　　DETAILS:

Do you do energetic things, like going for long walks, swimming, dancing, cycling etc.?
YES　　　　　　NO　　　　　　DETAILS:

Are there any problems with your partner or previous partners?
YES　　　　　　NO

Are you enjoying your sex life?

Are there any problems with your children?

Any other relationship problems?

Have any other members of the household got problems, and if so, who?

Have you kept fairly cheerful recently?

Have you felt depressed or low-spirited recently?

Have things been getting on your nerves much lately?

Have you been feeling tired during the day, even when you haven't been working very hard?

Is everything an effort?
YES   NO

Do you have trouble getting to sleep at night?
YES   NO   DETAILS:

Do you wake in the night or early morning and have trouble getting back to sleep?
YES   NO   DETAILS:

Anything else at all you can think of that might affect your health?

Do you feel in good health?
YES   NO   DETAILS

How did you hear about the Well Woman Clinic?

What made you decide to come to the Well Woman Clinic?

If we needed to contact you later, would it be alright to send a letter to your home?

FURTHER COMMENTS – GENERALIST

RESULTS OF TESTS

Possible tests	Tests wanted (tick)	Tests done	Results
Weight			
Height			
Urine test			
Vision			
Feet			
Blood pressure			
Haemoglobin			
Cervical smear			
Vaginal exam			
Breast exam			

ADVICE/ACTION

ADVICE WANTED ON
(TO BE COMPLETED WORKER)

ADVICE GIVEN BY WORKER

1.	
2.	
3.	
4.	
5.	

PROBLEMS IDENTIFIED WORKER	ADVICE GIVEN BY DOCTOR
1.	
2.	
3.	
4.	
5.	

FURTHER COMMENTS – DOCTOR

Number..............................

Name ....

Date of Birth...................................... Age.............

Address ....

....

....

General Practitioner ....

....

Date ....

INDEX

Alcohol dependency, 92–93
Antenatal care, 61–64

Beck Depression Inventory, 50–51
Biological determinism, 10, 13, 14, 40
Boston Women's Health Collective, 24

Carers, 17, 40
Childbirth, 57
Community care, 16–71
Coping behaviour, 85–90
Cost–benefit analysis, 173–175
Cost effectiveness, 172–175
Croxteth, 153
Culture, 9, 17

Dependency, 90–92
Depression, 85–86

Economic decision making, 167

Female doctors, 15, 139, 143, 150
Feminist, 20, 21, 23–24, 34–35, 51–52, 184
Feminist epidemiology, 18–19
Femininity, 11, 17
Florence Nightingale, 14, 41

Gender stereotyping, 39

Healers, 6
Health visitor, 111, 128, 139–140, 168–170, 180
Health week, 159
Health workers, 13
Hysterectomy, 39, 45–48

Labour, 64–68
Learned helplessness, 89–90
Life stressors, 86–87
Loss, 82

Mammography, 175–176
Marriage, 77, 80–87
Medical, 77, 80–87
Medical hegemony, 9
Medicine, 24, 29, 34–36
Mental health, 76
Midwife, 7, 16, 69–71
Motherhood, 83
Mothering, 17–18

National Health Service, 14, 16, 57, 97, 109, 119, 124, 165
Nature, 8–9
Nursing, 14–16, 39, 113, 181

Opportunity cost basis, 178–180
Option appraisal, 173–175

Perinatal mortality, 58–60
Personal control, 31–34
Philosophy, 8
Planning health care, 170
Postnatal, 69
Pregnancy, 29–31, 42, 44

Reproductive function, 10–13, 42–44, 46, 57

Screening, 176–178
Sexism, 15
Skill training, 93–95, 142
Social control, 12–13, 44
Stress, 77–80

Vauxhall, 162
Volunteers, 115, 118, 120–121, 125, 136, 163

Well women clinics
  establishment of, 97
  evaluation, 117–118, 126
  health questionnaire, 133
  models of, 100–103
  organisation, 134, 140, 145
  self help, 103–105, 143
  session, 132–133, 135

Rusholme, 138
values, 103
Withington, 129
Wythenshawe, 107
Witch, 67
Women's health courses, 123, 142, 157, 164
  movement, 23, 97, 108–110, 129
Women's movement, 10, 76, 97
Women's sexuality, 40–43, 45
World Health Organisation, 184